The INTENSE Trainer Program

The INTENSE Trainer Program

Nationally Certified Personal Trainer
Shane Chattin

iUniverse, Inc.
New York Lincoln Shanghai

The INTENSE Trainer Program

iUniverse books may be ordered through booksellers or by contacting:

iUniverse
2021 Pine Lake Road, Suite 100
Lincoln, NE 68512
www.iuniverse.com
1-800-Authors (1-800-288-4677)

ISBN-13: 978-0-595-36254-7 (pbk)
ISBN-13: 978-0-595-80699-7 (ebk)
ISBN-10: 0-595-36254-0 (pbk)
ISBN-10: 0-595-80699-6 (ebk)

Printed in the United States of America

Dedicated to Our Father

Contents

Introduction

The Intense Trainer Program is a thirty-day fat-loss program that was developed to dramatically enhance your quality of life. The key factor of the Intense Trainer Program is self-discipline. Without self-discipline, it is impossible to participate in any program, much less one of this nature. Self-discipline is the most overlooked aspect of any fat-loss program out there. If you do not have the discipline to complete a program, what good does it do to even start? You will never be able to stick with any program if you are unable to stay with it long enough to see results.

Once you start to see results, you will gain more motivation with every passing day. The psychological factors that affect dieting are the same factors that affect other areas of your life. This portion of the program will, without a doubt, have one of the biggest impacts on your life. When you gain a better understanding of the role self-discipline plays in your life, you will be able to understand the importance of establishing, strengthening, and maintaining self-discipline.

With this program, you will not have to guess what to do from one day to the next. Written out over thirty days, the program addresses the appropriate plan of action required to assist you in getting through each particular day. This is the element that will allow you to be successful, and take it day by day, instead of looking at the big picture and becoming overwhelmed. I am sure you have already imagined the way you want to look; it is now time to follow the steps required to make it happen!

The second factor that you must address to dramatically enhance your body is diet. Without a diet plan, you will never be able to consistently lose and keep off body fat. Once you have established the self-discipline needed to participate in a diet program, you will need to know what to eat. This program will teach you how to calculate the number of calories your body burns in a day.

Once you have established that number, you will know the maximum amount of carbohydrates and calories from other sources that you can eat in a single day. It is like a banking system—you will be given a number that you cannot go over, as well as a number that you cannot fall under.

Most people think that all they have to do to lose all the excess body fat they want is to cut back the amount of calories they eat. The problem with this theory is that your body reduces the amount of calories it burns when it senses that food is being withheld. As a consequence, your metabolic rate drops, and you end up losing healthy muscle that burns a lot of calories. When you lose muscle, you do lose weight, because muscle weighs more than fat. Drastic calorie cutting does not help you lose more fat. In fact, you will actually gain more fat when you go back to a more flexible way of eating. I know you have seen that process happen time and time again.

The metabolism is a somewhat complex function that is fully accounted for by this program. The ability to manipulate this bodily function is going to maximize your fat-loss efforts. You will be able to sleep well at night knowing that you are losing the most amount of body fat in the shortest amount of time possible.

The third factor used in this program is exercise. Exercise is only achieved when you actually do it. Most diets say that you should exercise—but what kind of exercise?

Some fat loss programs like to skim over the importance of exercise, because the diet makers know that you are dealing with discipline issues, or you would not be purchasing their products. They want their programs to appear as easy as possible, so they can get you to purchase their product on an impulse. The easier the program appears, the easier it will be to convince yourself that you can do it. That is why so many offer a thirty-day money-back guarantee. They know you won't have enough discipline to send the product back for a refund. This program was not designed to get you to purchase it on an impulse—it was designed to get you serious results. Exercising will become one of your favorite daily activities once you have the energy and discipline to actually do it.

Self-discipline, diet, and exercise: all three of these elements are required in order to achieve intense results. You cannot have one without the other two. If you want to just diet, you will fail every time and be forced to live with a less-than-desirable body. If you just exercise, you will eventually fall away from that as well, because you are not seeing results. The only one that you will not fall away from once you achieve it is self-discipline.

Once you have self-discipline, you will be able to easily maintain both a diet and an exercise routine. The combination of all three elements is what makes up the Intense Trainer Program. The results you gain from this program will stay with you for the rest of your life.

True confidence is gained only through hard work and dedication. When you complete this thirty-day program, you will have experienced one of the most intense fat-loss programs ever designed. You will gain a confidence that can only be experienced by those who complete the program. You will come to know and trust yourself more than you could have ever believed possible.

On that note, get ready for one of the most intense journeys you will ever take!

PART I
Self-Discipline

Self-Discipline Fundamentals

I decided to start with self-discipline, because without this element, you will not be able to complete this thirty-day training program. I highly recommend you check with your doctor before beginning. Be certain that you are capable of completing this program safely. Once you have your doctor's consent, you will be able to proceed without interruptions; however, if you do experience any symptoms that feel uncomfortable, make sure to ask your physician for further instruction.

I feel safe assuming that self-discipline is probably not one of your strongest areas. It was one of my weak areas for years until I realized its importance. One definition of discipline is "training that corrects, molds, or perfects." This is very important, because self-discipline training is the most overlooked aspect of any fat loss program. Have you ever heard of any diet that started out by teaching you self-discipline?

I sure haven't, or I would never have had issues with my own weight. I was not blessed with a highly tuned metabolism. I would use food to soothe my stress and laziness to comfort my mind. This combination is the leading cause of obesity in the world today. It is a double whammy: you want to eat so you can feel better, and you want to be lazy so you can feel better. Both actions are a result of wanting to feel better.

The problem with feeling better through gluttony and sloth is that your health pays the ultimate sacrifice. When someone is in this state, it takes a major intervention to snap him or her out of it. When you purchase any diet program, it is an attempt to gain back that self-control. Unfortunately, most people fall back into their old habits before they are able to replace the negative habits with positive ones.

I am sure that when you picked up this program, you were attracted to it because it offers you the opportunity to lose a lot of fat in a short amount of time. The truth is that there are a lot of diets with which you can lose a lot of fat in a short period of time, as long as you stick with it. I have chosen the most aggressive diet to get the fat off, because I want to prove to you that you can do it.

After you've made it through this thirty-day program, the results you have achieved will last a lifetime. I assure you that controlling your body composition will be the last thing you will have to worry about. You will be free to focus on the things that really matter in your life. Mastering self-discipline is no different than mastering any other aspect of your life. Once you have it, you are free to look at obtaining other things that are important to you.

It is my hope that, by the end of this program, you will have the tools and the knowledge necessary to be set completely free from the hold that you have had on yourself. Every day, I will be training not only your body but also your mind. Without strength in both, you are destined to fail. Once you have a strong mind, your body will certainly follow. Your outer appearance will be a direct reflection of the person you have always wanted to be.

How many times in your life have you started a diet, only to fail before the completion of it? I am guessing that it has been multiple times. If you were lucky enough to find this program on your first attempt at dieting, God bless you. You have no idea how lucky you are. The truth is that the majority of the people reading this program have failed numerous times in the past.

If you are one of them, do not blame yourself for this unfortunate circumstance. I never had anyone who trained and conditioned me in the area of self-discipline, so for a long time, I was stuck in the same place as the rest of the world: wanting to look a certain way but for some reason unable to change. It does not matter how badly you want to lose the excess body fat. The fact is that if you are not strong enough to see it through, you are not going to succeed.

I want you to think of a time when you attempted to lose body fat and failed, then answer these three questions: What was the reason you failed? How many days were you able to stick with the program? Did you gain the weight back once you stopped following the diet? Those are the three questions I ask potential clients. Their answers allow me to see their maturity in their walk toward self-discipline.

If someone tells me that he or she was unable to stick to a diet, I want to know why. Most people will tell me that it was too strict; some tell me that they did not like the foods that were in the diet; and some told me that they just did not want to complete it. I have heard thousands of excuses, but they all have one thing in common: The individual did not have self-discipline and talked himself out of completing the program. That is the bottom line. Most people will come up with a thousand reasons why they cannot do something when, in truth, they simply lack self-discipline.

Now I'm going to shock you—I think it is great that you made up the excuses, because if you had not, you would not be reading this today. Your ego had to create a reason not to complete that diet, because if it did not, you would have given up and never attempted a diet again. Self-esteem is directly linked to self-discipline. When you strengthen your self-discipline, you enhance your self-esteem dramatically. The two are actually one and the same. The only reason one person has confidence and someone else does not is that the one person had the strength to get through his or her own weaknesses.

Every time you attempt to lose weight and fail, you damage your ability to have discipline. Your ego compensates for your weakness by creating an excuse for why you could not lose weight at that time. You will come up with explanations like, "I know I can lose weight if I really want to, but I just have too many things going on right now." This type of excuse is one of the most common, but trust me, there are thousands more.

When someone tells me why they cannot start a program, I fully understand what is holding them back. I do not start by telling a client about all of the fun exercises I'm going to have them do or about the flexible meal plan. I start by asking them a series of questions that lets them search for the answer. I can tell you anything in the world, and you will not truly hear me. But when I ask you a question that only you can answer, you are forced to listen, because you're the one searching for the answer. The process that is taking place while you're searching for that answer is called *understanding*.

When you are attempting to learn why you cannot stick to a certain diet, you are really searching for the answer. You are searching for the answer because you want to make a change. When people are happy with a certain area of their lives, they do not feel a need to change it. When you are searching for the reason why you continue to fail at every diet program that you have ever participated in, remember that it really does not matter why you have not been able to lose body fat in the past. The only thing that matters now is that you are willing to say that you need to change. Once you can do that, you will begin establishing self-discipline.

In order to establish self-discipline, you have to slow down long enough to understand why you are doing something. Most people who come to me wanting to lose weight begin with an enormous amount of enthusiasm. They really are excited about knowing that, for once in their lives, they are going to have that dream body that they have always wanted. Every client that I have ever trained started out with that kind of enthusiasm but soon realized that my program is not about lifting weights and running on a treadmill—it is about establishing self-discipline.

When you go into a diet with big expectations, you are basically holding your breath and hoping that the program will work. The more enthusiasm you have, the deeper the breath you take. Eventually, you have to come up for air, and when you do, you will realize that you failed the program. Any big risk you take in life usually involves faith; you have to first believe that it can happen before it will. If you really do not know whether you will complete an exercise program, you will be forced to take a deep breath and hope for the best.

True confidence comes from knowing that you do not have to psych yourself up to complete something. You will be able to fall back on your faith to carry you through the tough spots. If you believe in God, this program may be a lot easier for you. When you can draw on a strength that is greater than you, then you can share the majority of the responsibility you take on with your creator. When you have only yourself to rely on, you have to dig deeper for the energy it takes to deprive your body of something that it has been using to soothe stress and anxiety. In order for you ever to have true strength, you must first understand where that strength comes from. I am a Christian, but I will not be using my faith in Christ to persuade you one way or the other. The search for truth is unique to everyone, and I have dedicated this program to losing body fat, not expressing my personal beliefs.

Applying self-discipline is a fairly complex action. Everything you do in life requires some sort of discipline. If you have to finish a project for work or go to the doctor for medical treatment, you have to tell yourself ahead of time that you need to do it. Once you decide you need to accomplish something, you have two choices. You can take a defensive position and sit back and hope that it comes to you, or you can take an offensive position and just get it done.

Most people live their lives in a defensive position; they exert the least amount of energy possible in order to make it through the day. When you are exerting only enough energy to get you through the day, you will never be able to accomplish anything. You will live your entire life doing only what you have to do in order to get by. It is sad to see people living their lives in this way, but most people are not even aware they are doing it. They have gotten so consumed by their negative past experiences that they are struggling to stay afloat. When you feel like you can be beaten, something very destructive happens inside your mind. Instead of looking at all the things you can accomplish, you are forced to look at all of the things you cannot do. This destructive process may already be affecting your life, if only in a very subtle way. If you are not able to do something when you say you are going to do it, you probably have a pretty good indication that you are struggling with this problem. Think about it. Why haven't you been able to lose body fat in the past?

Through self-discipline, you are going to crush the negative ideas you have about your ability to accomplish something. I will start you out with very simple tasks and build you up to very difficult ones. I will never ask more out of you than I know you are capable of doing. When I want to put muscle on someone's body, I do not start him off lifting four hundred pounds. I build him up slowly, step by step. As he gets stronger, he will be able to lift more weight and create more muscle.

When you start a diet plan, you have to do the same. You have to start off small and build your way up. Most diets recommend starting strict and tapering off once you get closer to your goal weight. I disagree. When you first start a program, you need to be able to win in order to get stronger. If you fail, you end up twice as far back as when you first started.

I learned a lot about building confidence from watching boxers and race-horses. They both share the same principle—they start out easy and work their way up, step by step. A boxing trainer can have one of the most talented fighters in the world under his instruction, and the trainer will still choose easier opponents until he feels that the fighter has built up enough real confidence to win the tougher fights. Think about it: that fighter had the ability all along to beat the tougher opponents. But the trainer knew his fighter did not have the confidence, so the trainer would only let him fight opponents that the trainer knew he could beat.

True confidence is achieved only by accomplishing something that you set out to do ahead of time. The same concept applies to racehorses: a racehorse starts out running against easier horses so that the horse can build up its spirit and confidence. The horse has the physical ability all along, but without the confidence, it cannot win.

If that horse and boxer had been beaten early, they would have never been able to realize their full potential. It doesn't matter how strong they are. If they believe that they can be beaten, they will never be able to maximize their own natural ability. Their trainers need to have them win before helping them improve. When I train someone whose self-esteem has been largely depleted, I do just that. I start by having her do things that I know she will not fail at. Once I know that she can handle more, I give her more to do. It usually does not take long before a client tells me that I am not working her hard enough. I love it when that happens, because I know she is starting to trust her own abilities. I have had the honor of training some of the most mentally tough individuals in the world. It never ceases to amaze me what someone can do when they have true confidence.

True confidence and false confidence are two different things. The ego is responsible for building false confidence, and you are responsible for building true confidence. Understand that the ego is used as the first step in building confidence. Most people have a negative perception of the role the ego plays. Without the ego, you would not be able to accomplish anything. The ego tells you that you can accomplish something when everyone else tells you that you cannot. Now it is up to you to actually do it. There are a lot of people who rely on their egos to do all of the work and expect to gain confidence from something just because they believe that they can do it. The person who speaks from true confidence knows that they can accomplish something, because they have already done it. They can look back and say, "Yeah, I know I can do it, because I already did it." That is true confidence. There is a huge difference between people who think they can do something and people who know they can do something.

One's outward appearance does not always match what lies underneath. I can recognize true confidence immediately. You know that you have true confidence when you are able to give someone an honest answer about what you can and cannot do. If someone asks me whether I can dramatically enhance his or her physique in a month, I can respond, "Yes," quite easily, because I have done it many times before.

Have you ever noticed that of all the many experts out there, very few have actually accomplished what they are teaching? A personal trainer who tries to convince people that they are going to lose weight could not be speaking from firsthand experience if the trainer has never had to diet a day in his or her life. You know that the people they are talking to are asking themselves, "What does this person know about weight loss? He has been thin all of his life!" If you do not speak from firsthand experience, you will have to rely on secondhand knowledge. A doctor who spends ten years in college does not have the confidence of a doctor who has been practicing medicine for twenty years. The doctor who is fresh out of college goes by only what he or she learned from secondhand knowledge. That is why doctors have to complete an internship. It is crucial that they are able to practice what they learned and put it into action. Those doctors will then be able to speak from firsthand experience and will have the confidence to make clear diagnoses.

This applies to personal trainers as well. A personal trainer may have learned in college what to do to help someone lose body fat, but it is not until he or she actually puts it to use and changes people's lives that he or she can speak from firsthand experience. This program is designed to give you true confidence by establishing self-discipline through firsthand experience, not secondhand knowledge.

When you start this program, you will be so focused on strengthening your self-discipline that you will forget about the major transformation your body is going through. You would not believe how many times I hear people tell me that they did not think that this program was going to be so easy. The only reason it was easy for them was that they stayed focused on self-discipline, not how much they wanted to eat.

Once you get the first week under your belt, everything starts to get a lot easier—not because your diet changes but because you have taken back the control that was stripped from you at some point in your life. This program will put you in a zone that can only be experienced by those who complete it. I promise you that the results are permanent. I do not care how much you want to sabotage yourself after you complete this program, it just will not happen. You will already know that you are capable of taking back control of your body, and no one can take that from you—not even you! Remember that once you have achieved something, you will always know that it is possible to do it again. That is real confidence.

In the next section, I will discuss the things you have succeeded at in your past, and show you how to use those successes for fuel. I have had people tell me that they have never succeeded at anything in their lives. This simply is not true, because if you are alive, you have succeeded at something.

Establishing self-discipline will be the foundation of everything you do from this point forward. After reading the next section, you will gain a better understanding of how to establish that self-discipline.

You will not actually do the exercises until you start the program. The program starts only after I have explained why I will have you do certain things in the program. If you do not understand the importance of what you are doing, then it is more than likely that you will not be motivated to do it.

Now that you have a better understanding of the importance of discipline, let's get started.

Establishing Self-Discipline

The first step in establishing self-discipline is believing that you will be able to do so. Every action in life starts out with a belief. Confidence comes from being able to apply that belief to an action and achieve a noticeable outcome.

A belief has three stages that it must go through before it produces a noticeable outcome. The first stage of a belief starts when you are able to say out loud what it is you believe in. The moment you say that you believe in something is the moment your mind starts to search for support for that belief. When you say that you believe you will have self-discipline, you are going to have to find reasons why you are going to have self-discipline. The moment you say you believe that you are going to be successful, you are going to have several different thoughts as to why you will be successful or why you will not be successful. How you address these thoughts will determine whether that belief gets a chance to take root. If you say that you believe you're going to be successful, but all you can think about is why you will not be, you will never get the opportunity to be successful.

Your mind operates in this way because it is a self-defense mechanism that keeps you safe, but this mechanism can also limit your opportunities. If you decide that you want to run out into oncoming traffic, there is a part of you that is going to say, "No, don't do it, or you'll get killed." That is a very healthy function of the mind. When you state that you believe you will lose body fat, and the first thought that pops into your head is that you cannot lose body fat, because you have already attempted to lose body fat in the past and failed every time. You have to address those limiting beliefs. If you do not correct those beliefs, you will continue to fail at losing body fat until they are corrected.

When you establish self-discipline, you are basically overpowering and removing old, limiting beliefs. If you are not able to overpower a belief that tells you that you cannot do something, then you can trust me when I say that you will never do it. Every thought that does not support your belief has to be removed so that you can accomplish your goals. As long as you continue to give in to your old negative beliefs, you will continue to be controlled by them. The important thing to remember is that the first step in correcting a negative belief is to physically speak your new desired belief out loud.

The second stage of developing a belief is defending your belief. When the thought pops into your head about all of the times you have failed in your past, you have to answer it with truth. The negative thought that pops into your head is none other than doubt. You have to eliminate doubt in order to establish a belief.

When you say that you will lose body fat and look great, and you do not have any negative thoughts pop into your head that tell you differently, you will know that you are heading in the right direction. The only thing stopping you from having what you want in life is *you*. This is a very humbling realization, but once you take responsibility for your own actions and quit blaming everyone else for your mistakes, you will start to establish self-discipline.

Most individuals do not pay close enough attention to their own thoughts. People become uncomfortable when they realize just how much junk goes into their head in one day, so they just stay fully associated and never take a good look at their lives. Some clients have told me that they do not want to look at their own lives because it will depress them. Obviously, if you are not able to take an honest look at your own actions, it will be very difficult for you to establish true confidence. You gain confidence when you stand up to those negative thoughts that interrupt your attempts to reach your goals.

If you are participating in a low-carb diet, and all you can think about is bread and pasta, you are going to fail the diet at some point. Remember, establishing self-discipline starts with your ability to believe that you can do it. That is why you have to work on your belief in yourself before you can move on to gaining the more complex aspects of self-discipline. The ability to defend your belief in yourself comes from being able to focus your thoughts on the things that support your belief.

The third and final stage of a belief is putting a belief into action. A belief is not a true belief until you have put it into action. It is very easy to fool yourself into believing that you can do something, but it is an entirely different story when you actually have to do it. I do not trust anything that I cannot see or experience firsthand. If someone tells me something, I do not truly believe him or her until I can see it for myself. That is a very natural function of a belief: a belief is not a belief until it produces a noticeable outcome.

When someone says they believe they can do something, they are only speaking in theory until they can actually do it and say, "There, I did it!" True confidence can only come from past success. If you tell me that you are going to walk up a flight of stairs, you are speaking in theory. It is impossible for you to know for sure that you are going to be able to walk up those stairs. You could fall and break your leg halfway up the stairs—or worse, you could have a heart attack and die halfway up. These are extreme examples, but you cannot deny the truth in them. True confidence can only come once you have climbed those stairs and said, "See, I told you I could climb those stairs!" You had to put that belief into action before you could speak from confidence.

Theories and assumptions are essentially the same. When you theorize something, you are relying on past experience to assume that if you do "A," you will get "B." You can climb those stairs with confidence, because you have climbed possibly thousands of stairs in your life and you feel safe assuming that you can do it again. The only variable is doubt. If you had not believed that you could climb the stairs, you could not have done it.

Right now, think of at least one thing that you said you were going to do and then actually did. Was that one thing something large, or was it small? The larger the accomplishment, the more confidence it will generate for you. The secret to achieving something big is to start out with something small and then allow it to snowball. The reason it is so easy to become consumed by the things going on in your life is that you are missing the smaller pieces.

When you stay focused on your goals long enough, you will eventually be able to accomplish them. It is *The Tortoise and The Hare* fable all over again. I would much rather have a strong foundation for a project and take longer to complete it than to gain massive success all at once, and place myself in a position where someone can pull out the rug from underneath me.

For example, when you start a new diet all at once, you may go and buy all of the foods you think you will be able to eat. Then a couple of days later, if even that long, you cheat. At that point, you cannot see the sense in eating all that healthy food if you have already wrecked your diet, so it sits and collects mold until you throw it out. This may not have happened to you yet, but it is a sad part of dieting for many. If this has happened to you, what happened is that you started out with the best of intentions but did not establish a strong enough foundation to complete it. The first step in laying your foundation is establishing self-discipline. Once you have poured your foundation, you are ready to start building.

The first thing to do to establish your foundation is to find out why you have failed at dieting in the past. Once you know the cause of your previous failures, you will be able to remove that cause once and for all. You have possibly developed hundreds of reasons to not lose body fat, but more than likely, only a handful of these reasons are true.

Most of the excuses I hear are secondary to the actual problem. When people tell me they are just too busy or that they do not have enough time to diet, I already know the source of that negative belief. When people tell me that they got stressed out and had to eat something to make themselves feel better, I know the source of that negative belief. When people tell me they just cannot lose weight no matter what they do, I know the source of that belief as well.

What I want to do is to allow you to see the main reason for your past failure, instead of the secondary reason. You may have several excuses you want to use, but if you take enough time to really think about it, I am certain you will see that every excuse can be traced back to one of the following problems:

Problem 1: If you have attempted to diet and felt overwhelmed by everything you had to do to maintain the diet, you are suffering from the first negative belief: that you have to focus entirely on what you eat. Your mind only thinks about food. However, one of the most important elements in completing a diet is not to focus on food at all. If all you can think about is eating only a certain type of food or about all of the things that you cannot eat, guess what? You will spend the majority of your day thinking about how limited you are by that diet.

The ability to control the direction of your thoughts is one of the first steps in establishing self-discipline. You will never be able to control the thoughts themselves, but you will be able to control the direction of them. For example, I do not want you to think about the color red. I said, do not think about the color red. Why did you think about the color red?

You cannot control what goes into your mind, but you can direct it once it is inside. If you see someone eating one of your favorite fattening foods, you cannot stop that image from going into your mind. However, you can decide to stop thinking about it and focus on the goal of sticking to your diet. This problem is the most common reason why someone fails on a diet program. If you cannot get your mind off the things that tempt you, you will feel like you are depriving yourself of something. When that happens, you are in the fast lane toward failure. If you can redirect that thought before it gains momentum, you can secure the belief that you will stick to your diet and that you will be just fine.

The more you allow yourself to think about the things that go against your belief, the further you get from that belief. When that happens, you end up so far from your belief that you forget what you were attempting to do in the first place. In that scenario, it would be only natural to feel that dieting requires a lot of energy and attention. But when you can immediately redirect the negative thoughts, you can diet with ease. Do not worry; your newly established self-discipline will be there to keep you on track, but it will require conscious effort.

Problem 2: The second most common reason people fail at dieting is stress. Stress arises when you feel that the circumstances surrounding your life are out of your control. This is a very simple obstacle to overcome, so we will begin there. The first thing to understand is that you do not have control over anything in your life. Take the example of climbing that flight of stairs. You did not know whether you could climb it until you actually did. No one can say for certain that something will happen, because they do not know. They are relying on the assumption that because they have done something before, they will be able to do it again. We have already established that you can only gain confidence from something that you have already accomplished, but even then, you still do not know if it will happen again.

People become stressed when they assume they should know in advance what to do in certain situations. How could you ever know in advance if the decisions you make are right? How do you know that the reason something failed was because it had to fail in order to set up the next step in your life? By nature, people are so power hungry that they feel they have to control every element of their lives.

This is an important topic, because you will deal with it again when you begin to strengthen your self-discipline. The more you can do, the more you will think that you have control. I do not care how disciplined you are—you will never have complete control of the things around you. One of the most important things to remember is that even when you have reached an amazingly high level of self-discipline, you will still never have complete control. This is where faith comes into play. You cannot have true confidence if you feel that you are in control of everything around you. If you think that you are in control of everything around you, you are still listening to your ego, not to reality. It would not be hard for you to think about all of the times that you believed a certain thing would happen and yet it did not. You are only lying to yourself if you feel that you have control over anything and everything. This is a very humbling realization, but once you are able to realize this, stress will no longer have a hold on you. You will come to realize that all you can do is what your mind will allow you to do.

This takes us back to the color red. The more times I tell you not to think about that color, the more times you think about it. Realizing that no one is in control of the things around them is a very uncomfortable experience for some. But that realization is absolutely necessary in order for you to establish self-discipline and overcome the stresses in your life.

Problem 3: The third problem is the most dangerous of all three, because it is the belief that that no matter what you do, you will not be able to lose body fat.

This belief is the most destructive of the three, because it indicates that all hope is gone. At that point, your self-esteem has been completely depleted, and all hope is lost. At least when you are giving excuses, you still feel that you are capable of losing the fat; you just have a reason why you cannot do it at that particular time. When you say to yourself that you cannot do something at all, you are imprisoned by that belief. You will not be able to overcome that belief until you have reestablished hope. The good news for you is that there is still some hope inside you, or you would not be reading this right now.

The person who completely lets go will never be brought back, but if you are still searching for an answer, do not fear; you still have the ability to get that fat off, and you have taken the right direction in order to make that happen. I like to refer to discipline as a balloon. The more you blow into it, the weaker it gets until it eventually pops. The secret to not popping the balloon is not to blow in it. The more reasons you have that you cannot do something, the more air you are putting into that balloon. Eventually, you will have blown so much air into it that it has to pop. When that happens, all hope is lost. You have no idea how lucky you are still to have the ability to search for an answer to your fat-loss issues.

This brings us to an important point. If you want to have self-discipline, you will have to accept the responsibility that comes along with it. When you were weak and unable to stick to something, you could always use that as your excuse. But once you truly obtain self-discipline, there are no more excuses. You will know that you are capable of accomplishing a desired goal. That is why you cannot take back self-discipline once you have it—what is there to give back? You already know from experience that you can discipline your thoughts in order to get a desired outcome. That will be a fact, and it will permanently disable the belief that you cannot do something. For the first time in your life, you will be able to state, with confidence, that you can complete a task. When you combine the ability to take responsibility for your actions and the ability to understand that you cannot control all of the circumstances around you, you are going to be prepared for the next step in discipline.

Now that we have addressed and discovered some of your old limiting beliefs, we will decide what you want to do with them. You have two choices when you want to discard an old negative belief. The first thing you can do with it is pretend that it never even existed. This is the most common choice, because most people want to choose the path of least resistance. The second alternative is to use that old belief as fuel to prepare for your new positive belief. You do this by establishing what you do not want and looking toward what you do want. This is better known as motivation.

When you are focused only on the things that you do not want to happen, those things will be drawn to you. They are drawn to you because the things that you think about are what make up your future. If you think about the things that you do want in life, those things are going to draw closer to you as well. If you have not been able to experiment with this idea before, I encourage you to do so now. You need to fully experience the reality of understanding that your thoughts are what guide your actions and ultimately create your future. You are what you focus on. I know that is easy to say but much harder to actually apply.

This takes us back to the ability to direct thought. When you see something that does not support your belief, goals, or ideas, you need to get away from it. When you are establishing self-discipline, you are doing just that: you are establishing the foundation of your thought process.

In the next section, we will be discussing strengthening self-discipline. When you strengthen your ability to withstand the temptation that goes along with having discipline, you will be able to start putting more responsibility on yourself. But for now, we just want to establish the belief that you will be able to do it. The most common mistake people make when they begin building their confidence is to put themselves in a compromising position that jeopardizes their ability to withstand temptation. It would be like me going into an ice-cream store the day after I start a low-carbohydrate diet. I would be setting myself up to fail.

When you first start any disciplined program, you have to make it as easy as possible. If you do not, you will only be setting yourself up for failure. I have made this mistake several times in my life before I realized what I was doing to myself. Everyone wants to think that they have enough strength to fight off the temptations, but it is an entirely different story once you fail. I want your foundation to be strong, so I am going to eliminate as many of your distractions as I can during the first week of this program.

I am going to move you along at a pace that you can handle. Whether you think you are strong or believe that you are weak, I start all of my clients out at the foundation and build them up from there. How quickly you accelerate depends on your willingness to follow directions. The ability to follow directions is another very important element of this program. If you want to continue the way you are living now and not make any changes, this program is not for you. I am hoping that I have scared off the majority of the weak people with the title of this program. If you did not have the desire to lose body fat, you would not have purchased a program of this nature.

Whether you feel you do not have enough time to diet, you feel too stressed, or you still feel like you cannot lose weight, you have to make the decision right now whether or not you are going to stick to this program. You will not get anything out of the rest of this program if you are not willing to accept the fact that you must first believe that you are going to succeed. Right now, do you feel that you have what it takes to stick with this program for thirty short days? If not, you really need to take a good look at why you are not able to move forward.

You must first realize that if you say you are going to do something, you are going to do it. For the next ten minutes, I want you to think only about the things that you have done right in your life. I do not care how small they are. You could be proud of the fact that you were smart enough to realize that you needed help and picked up this program. If that is the only thing you can think about, use it. Think about it over and over again. It is very possible that you have lived so many years looking at what you could not do that you have not been able to see what you could do. There is not a person alive who cannot establish self-discipline; you just have to get serious and do it.

Once you believe that you will be able to complete this program, you will be ready to move on to the next step. The next step will involve strengthening your self-discipline. Once you start to strengthen your self-discipline, you will be able to enjoy many of the benefits that come along with discipline. I hope that you have been able to establish the true reasons why you have had problems in your past, and I encourage you to stay committed and complete this program. Just make sure that you really believe that you will be able to do it. Once you have accomplished this, you are ready for the next step!

Strengthening Self-Discipline

Now that you believe that you will be able to successfully complete this program, we are ready to take that belief to the next level. Self-discipline goes through several stages as it matures. When self-discipline is in infancy, you will have to be very careful not to place yourself in a situation that is going to tempt you. If you allow even a small backslide in the beginning of this program, it will have a disastrous result.

Discipline operates on a set of parameters, as does any solid belief. If your goal is to complete this program, anything that goes against this program is outside the parameters of that belief. For example, if you commit to following a low-carbohydrate diet but later decide that one little piece of bread will not hurt you and so you eat just that one piece of bread, you will feel compelled to eat another piece of bread, because you have already gone against the diet once. You tell yourself that it will not hurt you to eat another piece, because you can get back on track the next day. Now you eat the entire loaf, because you want to get your fill before you withhold carbohydrates from yourself again. That is one of the most common scenarios of fat-loss failure.

The reason you do this is a lot more complex than you may think. There is a reason why your body feels the need to overeat. Whenever you think that you are depriving yourself of something, your body is going to have a reaction. It is only natural to have this reaction, because if you were still living in the days when food got scarce at certain times of the year, your body would have to store up extra body fat in order to make it through the tough times. It is a biological function that tells your body that something is missing and must be stored. When food does become available, you are going to overeat in order to compensate for the times your body had to go without.

You are the only one who knows when you are going to be able to eat your next meal. Your body is just doing its job. That is why self-discipline goes against the natural process of your body. Anything that goes against your body's natural process is going to require work. It is sometimes hard for someone to understand why he or she cannot just do something. You want to lose fat, so just lose the fat.

It sounds simple, but there must be something going on that will not allow you to do it.

When you are strengthening discipline, you are training and conditioning your body to withstand the temptations that go along with withholding something that you want and perhaps feel that you need.

If you love chocolate cake but are actively seeking to lose body fat, you logically understand that the piece of cake is not going to help you lose the fat. But when you are in the active state of wanting something, you really do not care. You just want that piece of cake. We are going to be training and conditioning that state. You are always going to submit to the things that you want more. If you want to eat chocolate cake more than you want to lose weight, you are going to eat that cake. The stronger desire will always win out.

Focus is the only tool you will be able to use to remedy this problem. When you realize that you will be able to have that casual piece of chocolate cake once you have reached your goals, it will be a lot easier for your body to understand why it is going through all of that discomfort. The most common error people make when they are in that wanting state of mind is feeling they are going to have to withhold those foods for the rest of their lives. That is not true, because it is only for a very short period of time in your life.

When you put it into context, it is fairly simple to see that all you have to do when you are being tempted to eat something that goes against your diet is to understand that you will be able to have it once your diet is complete. The ability to think clearly when you are dealing with an urge that goes against your belief is the main target we attack when strengthening self-discipline. If you are not able to redirect that thought before it has time to cause a physical action, you will continue to fail. In order for you to understand what state you are in when you feel like going against your belief, you must first be able to identify it.

Right now, I want you to think of a time when you were really committed to doing something. I want you to have a very clear image of what it looked like to you. Once you have that clear image, I want you to notice any sounds that may have been audible at the time. Maybe there were negative thoughts that were in your head, or perhaps you just felt compelled to act on what it was you wanted to do. The clearer the image is, the more beneficial it is going to be for this exercise.

Maybe you felt the overwhelming urge to go out and do something nice for someone, or maybe you decided to do something really nice for yourself. It really does not matter what it was that you were committed to do, just as long as you completed it.

Now that you have been able to form a really clear image of what you felt like when you were committed to doing something, I want you to develop a clear image of a time when you thought you were committed to doing something but, after a short period of time, you quit. Is this image clearer than the first one? If it is, we need to work on bringing more awareness to the times you have succeeded at doing something that you set out to do in advance.

The days of feeling sorry for yourself are over; it is now time to concentrate on the fact that you are going to be able to do the things you set out to do. The only things that I want you to concentrate on are the things you know you can do. If you have the ability to sweep your floors, do it. If you have the ability to go for a walk, do it. Any form of action that you take can be utilized as fuel to feed your ability to have self-discipline. The only problem you have had in the past is that you have not given yourself enough credit. The only reason I am able to strengthen your ability to have discipline is that I am going to shine a light on the things that you were probably oblivious to before. It is a very hard task to give yourself credit for doing something, because more than likely, you can think only about the things that you are not able to do. That is going to stop right here.

I could not care less how many things you feel that you cannot do. I just want to hear about the things that you *can* and *will* do. You are not going to be able to establish massive self-discipline overnight, but you will over a month. If you are still not convinced that you really want self-discipline, you need to go back to the last section and start over.

Now that we have established that you are not going to dwell on the things that you cannot do, it is time to focus on the things that you can do. I want you to list ten things that you will be able to accomplish today. It does not matter how simple they are. You just have to write them down. If you do not write them down, this exercise is not going to do you any good.

Remember, we have not started the actual program yet, because we are still discovering the role that self-discipline plays. This is not a test, but it is important that you do it. When you are able to write out a list of the things that you need to do, and you do everything on the list, you will get to experience the first step in strengthening self-discipline.

The act of committing to something on paper is a very powerful tool. Just make certain the ten things you list are very simple, such as brushing your teeth or combing your hair, for example. When you are first starting out, they can be things that you know you are going to do anyway. Even though these are things that you would normally do anyway, once you write them on paper and know that you have to do them, you may find that the simple little things you do in a day actually require discipline in order to get them done. If you need to go to the grocery store, do not write just "Go to the grocery store." Write down what you need to purchase at the grocery store. If you have to go to work, write down what you need to accomplish at work.

This may seem tedious at first, but there are several reasons why you are doing this. This is one of the most powerful exercises you can do to start bringing awareness to the things that you actually accomplish in a day. This is going to change the weaker areas of your beliefs that have been limiting you up to this point. It is easy to do things when you really do not need to, but it is an entirely different story when you need to do them. Something shifts in your mind when an action changes from being something that you want to do into something that you need to do.

When you want to do something, you are making a decision based on pleasure, and when you need to do something, you are making a decision based on necessity. The problem you may experience with dieting is that you may not have the want or need to diet. This is extremely important, because the majority of people starting a diet do not have the proper want or need established. When you go from the state of wanting something to needing something, the same belief has to be in place. If you just want to lose weight, but you do not feel that you need to lose weight, you are going to fail the diet, because the first time you are tempted to quit, your mind will switch states.

When this happens, your need to lose weight will not be there, and you will have no problem quitting the program. I cannot stress enough how important it is to have your mind in agreement with your goals. Your mind cannot be divided. It has to be at one with your decision in order to be disciplined. You must first have the want, and then you will have to create the need. Everything you do in life is directed by want and necessity. The power of wanting something will always be stronger than the power of necessity when it comes to self-discipline, because self-discipline is a conscious choice, and need is a required action that has to happen in order to survive. When you decide to establish that you not only want to diet, but you that need to diet, you are ready to take the next step.

Right now, I want you to think of a time in your life when you really wanted something. I want you to develop the clearest image possible. Notice any thoughts that you may have had. The important thing is that you are able to feel the way that you felt when you wanted that particular something. How did you feel when you wanted it? Did you feel anxious about obtaining it? Did you feel afraid that you were not going to obtain it? Or did you just feel in awe of the fact that you wanted it? Make certain that you are utilizing the strongest memories possible. I want you to really remember what it felt like to really want something.

Now that you have a really clear image of what it is that you wanted, I want you to imagine a time when you really needed something. I want this image to be just as clear as the wanting image. Pay special attention to the way you feel. Do you feel any different than you did when you wanted something? If so, what are the differences? The most common difference is certainty. When you feel like you want something, you will often feel uncertain about what to do. Your actions will be indecisive, and your ability to make a decision will be impaired. If you feel that you need something, you know that you do not have a say in the matter. A need is something that has to be done in order to ensure survival. When you feel that you have to do what you have to do in order to survive, you just do it. The ability to just do something comes when you are able to create the feeling that you need something, not merely that you want it. Many times, the only reason you were able to obtain something that you wanted is that you were able to distort that want into a need.

Now we are going to convert your ability to want to diet into a need. Once we do this, you are going to be able to take a big step toward strengthening your self-discipline. The first thing you will need to do is write down the reasons why you feel that you want to diet. I want you to list at least ten different reasons that you feel dieting will create pleasure in your life. Once you have written down ten different reasons why you want to diet, I want you to list at least ten different reasons why you feel you need to diet. This may take you a while, but you need to do it, because it is essential to your success in this program.

Without the ability to know why you are doing something, you will always get defeated when your mind switches from a want to a need. Now that you have a better understanding as to why you are going to be dieting, you are ready to move forward. You will be able to rely on both your wants and your needs. When you are feeling good, you will be able to think about all of the great things you will be able to do when you are healthy, and when times get tough, you will be able to fall back on the fact that you need to continue dieting for your health. You will be working both urges in the direction that leads to stronger self-discipline.

Are you able to recall a time when you wrote out a list of all of the things you needed to do but got sidetracked and didn't complete all of them? Every time you say you are going to do something and don't do it, you fall further away from being able to strengthen your self-discipline. You have to understand that if you don't do what you say you are going to do, you will be unable to take yourself seriously. Once you are able to start accomplishing what you say you are going to do, self-discipline strengthens itself. You do not need to consciously train self-discipline. When you complete the exercises in this program, discipline has to strengthen itself. You will not need to think about what you should be doing, because you will already be doing it.

When you write out a list of the reasons you want to do something, as well as the reasons you need to do something, you will establish the parameters of your daily goals. When you stick to the plan you created, discipline will handle itself. It is hard for some people to grasp this concept, because they know that things will pop up and make it more difficult to stay with the plan. When something unexpected comes up in your life, you will always have the ability to formulate a new plan. This is where taking responsibility for your actions comes into play.

Strengthening your self-discipline combines several factors into one formula that gets you results. When you combine the ability to believe that you can complete this program with the need and want to complete this program, nothing can stop you from doing it. Taking action is a result of developing a well-thought-out plan. If you just decide to wing it, you will never be able to give yourself enough credit for the things that you have done to obtain results.

It is important to keep in mind that self-discipline goes through several stages before it begins to mature. Every step has to be strengthened individually. If you attempt to just jump into self-discipline with everything you have, you will eventually get overwhelmed and fail. The only way you are going to be able to complete this program is to successfully complete one day of training at a time. If you think about having to do what you did on one particular day for thirty days, you are going to have serious doubts. Every day will have its own plan of action.

If you attempt to do too much at one time, you will only end up further behind than where you were when you first began. It is very natural to want to achieve everything all at one time, but it is impossible. Each day will set up the next, until you have built up an enormously large amount of confidence. If you ever wanted to know the secret to life, that is it: Start out with a strong foundation and build up from there. This will be the most utilized tool in the Intense Trainer Program. The power of being able to start out with little or nothing and turn it into something that can only be described by experience is something that you will never forget. Think about it. All you have to do is gain one little bit of confidence every day. Before you know it, you will have an abundance of ability. Please keep this in mind as you start to strengthen your discipline. It will require a certain amount of patience, but the wait will definitely be worth it.

Once you start to strengthen your self-discipline, you are going to run into some things that have to be dealt with. The first is self-control. Once you see how effective you really are, you are going to develop a certain amount of power. When this starts to happen, you have to be ready for the side effects that come along with power.

We touched on this in the last section, but the effects of strengthening your self-discipline are going to begin to come alive when you complete the exercises in this section. It is only natural to feel that you have control over the things around you when you see how much control you now have over yourself, but you must keep in mind that just because you have control over your actions, does not mean you have control over the actions of the people around you.

I cannot tell you how many times clients have gotten a major power trip once they started to realize their potential. For so many years, you have been pushed around by your own weaknesses, and for the first time in your life, you have some control. Most people end up overcompensating and creating a personal power monster. Eventually, they realize that they are miserable, because no one wants anything to do with them. They end up losing the majority of that power, because they begin to associate discomfort with having self-discipline. Your ego is your business, but when it may get to a point where it interferes with this program; I'll point out the signs that go along with overreacting to confidence. Some people are blessed with an amazing ability to balance themselves out; however, if you have had low self-esteem for the majority of your life, you are going to feel the need to exude some of that long-overdue confidence.

This is a very natural process, which takes place when someone finally gains the upper hand in his or her life, but it is important to remember that confidence can go just as quickly as it came. The fear of losing it is what will give you the ability to maintain it. In the next section, we are going to discuss the steps you will need to take to ensure that you are able to maintain the newfound confidence that you have established through strengthening self-discipline.

Maintaining Self-Discipline

Now that you have established the belief that you will be able to complete this program, and you have seen how we are going strengthen your self-discipline, it is time to discuss how to maintain that discipline once you have it.

The transformation that will take place over the next thirty days is going to be very intense. Whenever you experience a positive shift in your abilities to accomplish something, you will also have to deal with the worry that comes along with wanting to hold onto it. When you get to experience a life-changing transformation such as this, many things are going to change in your life.

One of the first things you are going to notice is the amazing amount of confidence that you have gained. When you have the resistance to temptation that comes along with self-discipline, you will have no other choice but to get stronger. When you have obtained confidence, you will be able to think clearly for possibly the first time in your life.

So many people think that in order to find out who they really are, they have to look deep within themselves. In order for you to be able to look deep within yourself, you have to be willing to let down your ego. When you lower your ego, you are opening yourself up to every negative thought that you have ever been exposed to. We need to take a closer look at what the ego's job really is. Without self-esteem, you will never be able to fight off the negative thoughts that are waiting to make sure you fail.

It is important to point out what the ego is and the role that it plays in your life. The ego has a lot of negative associations that come along with it. One of the biggest misconceptions about it is that people with an ego are usually "cocky" and "conceited." When you see someone who acts cocky and conceited, you see a person who is actually struggling with his self-esteem. When you are struggling to gain self-esteem, you end up overcompensating with physical action in anticipation of gaining what it is that you are actually wanting. This is one of the most common forms of false confidence.

The definition of ego is *self-esteem*. If you do not have self-esteem, you will never be able to have an identity. From the time you were young, you started to develop a personality. The decisions you make in life and the beliefs you hold are what make you who you are. If you did not have self-esteem, you would not have an identity.

I know a lot about this subject, because at one point in my life, I actually consciously lowered my self-esteem to a point where it was almost completely gone. I know what it feels like to experience this process firsthand. Luckily, I chose to do this, thinking that I would be enlightened. If I had not chosen to lower my self-esteem, I would not have been able to know what was causing all of the things that were happening in my mind. When someone suffers from depression, it is a direct result of having his or her ego depleted. I speak from experience when it comes to anything that is contained in this program. There is not one thing in this program that I have not experienced firsthand. Your self-esteem is more important than you could have ever possibly imagined.

The ability to choose is not something that you should take lightly. When you are depleted of self-esteem, you have to rely on what everyone around you tells you. You lose the ability to make your own decisions, and you will be forced to live your life for everyone but yourself. When you decide to take a look at your life, you have to do it with the intention of helping yourself. If you want to look at why you continue to fail at dieting, you have to do it in a constructive way. You should be observing your weaknesses only to help yourself.

I like to pose this question to clients before they take that honest look at their lives: When you are judging yourself, who is doing the judging? This is a very frightening question, if you really think about it. In order for you to judge your own life, you have to create another identity. How can you look at yourself when you are the one doing the looking? You cannot. In order for you to take an honest look at your life, you have to let your ego down to become disassociated, and take a look at yourself without being able to defend yourself. When you are disassociated, you are in a neutral position. You are not really judging; you are only watching. Many people think that this is enlightenment, but they are sadly mistaken. They are just experiencing a separation from their own identity. This sense of separation happens when you are able to separate your mind from your body.

Someone who has suffered a major accident will often experience this out-of-body feeling. It is a real function within the mind, and I assure you that you do not want to experience this feeling. I could give you a step-by-step guide to consciously walking to this state, but I never will. The side effects of this experience are often more than most people can handle. Your mind is a lot more fragile than you may think.

I hope that you are starting to get a better understanding of why you need to have self-esteem. Having self-esteem does not mean that you have an over exaggerated opinion about your self-worth. It means that you have the ability to choose who you want to be and what it is in life that you want to do.

People experience different forms of disassociation all of the time. When you are faced with a life crisis, you have to disassociate yourself from the scenario in order to cope. The ability to disassociate yourself from a certain event is a natural function, just as long as you are disassociating yourself for the good of your well-being.

An example of disassociating yourself for the wrong reason would be when you get angry and you want to do something that you know is not right. In order for you to be able to override your conscience, you have to be willing to disassociate yourself from the scenario. In order for you to cheat on a diet, you have to be willing to temporarily separate yourself from the belief that you want to lose weight. The secret to being able to maintain self-discipline comes from being able to stay fully associated. The ability to stay focused is the same ability that allows you to stay associated.

True confidence can only be achieved when you are fully associated. In order for you to be confident, you have to be willing to take the chance of failing. When you are disassociated, you are in a neutral position. You are just doing what you have to do in order to survive. If you are in a fully associated position, you are willing to take the chances that come along with living in an offensive position.

Remember that when you are disassociated, you do not have the ability to judge right from wrong. The only thing you can do is what you feel you need to do in order to survive. When you are associated, you have to take responsibility for your actions. If you attempt something and fail, you realize that you did not make the right decision in that circumstance. You learn from your mistake, and you walk away with more knowledge than you had before. When you are truly confident, you always have the ability to move on. This is a direct result of having self-esteem.

In order to have self-esteem, you are going to need energy. If you do not have enough energy, you will never be able to accomplish the things you want in life. The only reason you are able to accomplish anything is you have the energy to do it. When you say you are going to do something, and someone tells you why you will not be able to, it will take energy to defend the belief that you are actually going to do it. When your energy gets low, you end up turning on yourself.

Many of you reading this can understand this firsthand. When you set out to diet and lose all of the excess body fat, you will need enough energy to actually do it. Everyone likes to talk about physical energy, but few people look at the significance of mental energy. In order to have the energy to stick to your diet, you are going to have to be full of mental energy. Mental energy is the same energy that fuels your self-esteem.

Mental energy, like physical energy, requires fuel in order to operate. Every time you discipline yourself to accomplish something, you are refueling your mental energy. I use the term *mental energy* to describe the phenomenon of self-discipline. I do not care how much food you eat; the only way to refuel the energy I am referring to is by discipline.

I am certain that you have experienced firsthand how you feel when you over-eat. Most people feel somewhat miserable and sometimes require a nap in order to get through the rest of the day. The food you put into your mouth is not the same food that you will need to feed your mind—it is actually the exact opposite. When you withhold food from yourself, you will get to experience some of the best results. Once you get past the hunger pangs that come along with withholding food, the mind will actually prefer to think in starvation mode. There is a reason why people fast, and it is not to lose body fat. This program is going to put your body in a state that will be burning a lot of fat. When that happens, you are in the same state that someone experiences when they fast.

Everything in this program is centered around this one very important question: Why can't you lose the excess body fat? You know that there is no physical reason, so there must be a mental reason. The only reason you have not been able to lose excess body fat and maintain your results is that your mind is not allowing you to do so. The only reason your mind is not supporting you is that you are not providing it with the energy that it needs.

I encourage you to look a little deeper into what I just said. You have to understand how self-esteem works in order to maintain it. I wish I could tell you that there was a magic pill that would give you the ability to do anything you wanted to do in life, but there is not. You have to understand that you must be willing to take care of more than what is visible to the eye.

It is challenging for someone to understand what to do in order to maintain his or her mental energy. Self-discipline is an action that relies on understanding, not the things that can be seen with the eye. If you do the exercises in this program and you are able to understand why I am having you do them, you are successfully training a function of your body that you cannot see. When runners train, they are able to see their results by the times in which they complete their runs. When you train self-discipline, you are training a part of the body that cannot be observed by a stopwatch. It will only be measured by the results you receive. When you start to notice that you have enough energy to stay disciplined on your diet and exercise program, you are going to start to understand that there is more to self-discipline than what you may have previously believed.

When you have reached the level of self-discipline that allows you to accomplish anything you want, it will be difficult for you to imagine ever living without it. Believe it or not, you have always had self-discipline; you just have not been able to fully utilize it. Now that you are at a point where you realize that you have self-discipline, you really have to focus on not letting it go. Once you have gained high levels of self-discipline, you will always be able to fall back on that, but it will require regular maintenance.

The first thing you will need to do to ensure that you maintain your discipline is never to breach the boundaries that you set when you were establishing and strengthening it. You have to make sure that you always hold yourself in check, or self-discipline can slip away from you just as quickly as you received it. In order to make sure that you stay within your boundaries, it is important to stay organized. Organization is one of the most important aspects of maintaining your self-discipline. When you feel as if your life is getting out of control, it is usually a direct result of disorganization.

One of the great side effects of having self-discipline is the ability to stay organized. Do you feel better when your house is clean, compared to when it is dirty? Of course you do! The ability to stay organized comes with knowing how good it feels to have some control in your life. The more things that you can do to obtain this control, the stronger your self-discipline will become. If you have a clean vehicle and a clean house, that may be a pretty good indication that you have a really firm grip on your life.

I will never forget a job interview I attended once. The gentleman who owned the business was a former Green Beret in the army. I had a lot of respect for him, because I knew the level of discipline that was required in order to be in Special Forces. He did something that I have never heard any employer do before: In the middle of the interview, he asked to see my vehicle. I was a little puzzled at his request, but I went along with it anyway. As we walked outside, he told me that he could learn a lot about someone by the way they cared for their property. At that point, I was really hoping that I had not forgotten to clean out my truck. As we reached my vehicle, he first looked at the outside of the truck to see if I kept it somewhat clean. He then asked if I would mind opening the vehicle. I was really becoming concerned at that point. After looking inside my truck, he said that he was very impressed with how I maintained my vehicle. He stated that it reflected self-respect. I told him that I had several papers on my front seat and that I could not comprehend how he got that impression from looking into my vehicle. He responded: "I was not looking at your seats. I was looking at your floor mats." When he opened the vehicle, he had looked to see if I took enough time to vacuum my vehicle out.

The outer appearance of your life is a direct reflection of what is going on inside your mind. I hope that you are one of the lucky people out there who realize just how fortunate they really are, but if you are not, it is time to appreciate the things that you do have and take care of them. The more things in your life that are clean and organized, the easier it will be to maintain them.

I have always had to struggle with staying on top of organizing the things around me. Everyone has a flaw that challenges them. My biggest flaw for years was not being able to maintain self-discipline. I was the one who would hold my breath long enough to get what I wanted, but the first time I came up for air, I would lose it. I have had several different times in my life when I was in phenomenal shape, but I was never able to stay that way. I always had to have something motivating me. Once that motivation went away, so did my physique. I was only holding my breath long enough to get what I wanted, and then I would ring the bell and say, "I did it."

Motivation to do something is useless if you do not have the discipline to back it up. How many times in your life have you been extremely motivated to do something, but once you accomplished it, you decided that it really was not worth having? I can assure you that self-discipline will not disappoint you. When the going gets tough, you will have yourself to rely on, possibly for the first time in your life.

It is important for you to understand that not everyone will be able to complete this program. When you successfully complete this program, you will be among a very small group of people. Most people will never have 10 percent of the amount of self-discipline that you are going to have. You will not be the average person by any means. Have you ever heard someone criticize another person because that person did not have the ability that the first one had? That person has to criticize someone, because he or she is envious of the other person's abilities.

As you start to experience the gifts that come along with having confidence, there will always be someone who tries to bring you down. As long as you understand why they are behaving this way, you will be in a position in which your confidence cannot be shaken. The only time someone will have an effect on you is when you're not able to defend yourself. If someone tries to insult you, the easiest way of defusing them is to agree with them. You are using your intelligence to defeat their ignorance. The ability to maintain your self-discipline comes from understanding why people behave the way they do. When you are able to understand why someone behaves the way he or she does, you will no longer feel a need to judge that person. Instead of being offended, you will feel empowered by your ability to understand his or her actions. This is one of the most effective tools you will be using to maintain your results.

After you complete this program, some of your friends may tell you that you must have gone through some major transformation, because everything in your life appears to be going so smoothly all of the sudden. It is interesting how discipline has such a smooth look to people who do not have it. They look at your organized life and are amazed at how easy it looks. If this is not your life now, do not worry—it will be soon. You are still reading because you really want to change. Some people reading this have already quit. I admire you for having enough strength to stay disciplined long enough to read about the importance of what we will be doing. It takes patience and understanding to learn why you are doing something. The majority of the people who pick up this program want to jump right in and attempt to start the program without understanding why they are doing it. I hope that you will continue to stay focused and keep on reading. The next section will address why I am going to have you eat the way you will be eating.

Without the participants' ability to understand the importance of self-discipline, this program would not be successful. After you have completed this program, you will have a deeper understanding of the things that I have mentioned in this section. You have to remember to take this program one day at a time, and discipline will take care of itself. I hope that you now have a better understanding of why I will have you doing some of the things that you will be doing in the exercise portion of this program. If, for some reason, you begin to feel that you may be slipping away from your routine, make sure that you read this entire section again. I have placed a lot of information in this section, and the more times you read it, the better off you will be.

PART II
Diet

Dieting Fundamentals

The diet that I have selected for this program is without question one of the most intense diets on the market today. This program will be utilizing the two most effective elements available in order to ensure rapid fat loss. The first element of the diet that I have selected is part of a very low-carbohydrate diet. The second element I have selected is part of a controlled-calorie diet. When you combine these two elements, you have just created one of the most intense forms of dieting known to man.

You may have heard about the low-carbohydrate/low-fat diet debates that have been in the media. I have dedicated this section to clearing up a lot of the misconceptions about the different forms of dieting. I hope that you will be able to gain a better understanding of why you will be eating the way you will in this program. If you are unaware of the process your body will be going through as you participate in this program, it will be difficult for your mind to justify the need to do it.

My career has been centered around being able to guarantee results. In order for me to guarantee a client that I can get the excess body fat off his or her body by a certain amount of time, I have to know that what I am having them do is the most aggressive approach that I can take while maintaining his or her nutritional needs. When I started to research the body's ability to burn excess fat, I started with looking at what the body required in order to function properly. Once I knew what the requirements were, I started to work on maximizing as many alternatives as I could to ensure success while still maintaining the proper amount of nourishment for the body. This program takes losing excess body fat to the absolute limit. When you withhold carbohydrates from your body and restrict the amount of calories that are going into it, you create a condition that will allow you to lose the most amount of body fat in the shortest period of time.

In order to properly distinguish the differences between a low-fat diet and a low-carbohydrate diet, we need to look at them separately. When you participate in a low-fat diet, you are limiting the amount of fat that is consumed by your body. The theory is that by withholding fat from your diet, you will allow your body to burn the excess body fat.

When you reduce the amount of fat your body consumes, you are reducing the number of calories that go into your body. One gram of fat contains nine calories. This is the highest calorie-to-gram ratio of all of the nutrients. One carbohydrate contains only four calories. That is less than half of the amount of calories in one gram of fat. It does not take a rocket scientist to figure out why you can lose weight on a low-fat diet. You are simply not consuming as many calories.

Everything about weight loss centers around the amount of calories you consume compared to the amount of calories your body burns. This is the simplest way of looking at it. I have a problem with low-fat dieting, which is why I did not select it for this program: when you are supplying your body with an abundance of carbohydrates, your body is going to choose carbohydrates as the predominant fuel source.

I do not want you to have carbohydrates as your primary fuel source, because I want you to be burning as much stored body fat as possible. Every carbohydrate you consume gets utilized for energy before stored fat. It may surprise you that I am a low-fat dieter, because I love bread and pasta. The low-fat approach is what suits my tastes over the long haul, but it is the low-carbohydrate dieting that gets me the results. If I feel as if I am starting to gain body fat, I know that it is a result of providing too many carbohydrates to my body. Once I cut back the carbohydrates, I quickly lose the excess fat. This diet was not designed for you to be on it the rest of your life. It was designed to get all of the excess body fat off in the shortest period of time possible.

The reason most diets fail is that people are not able to see quick enough results. This program is intense in every sense of the word. You are basically taking total control over your body, and how you choose to eat after you have done that will depend on your individual desires. You will be able to maintain your body any way that you see fit once all of the fat is off.

When you look at low-carbohydrate diets, you have to understand why people usually choose to do them. The most common reason people are drawn to a low-carbohydrate diet is that they want to be able to eat more food and still lose weight. There are many problems associated with that theory. When you reduce your carbohydrate intake, you reduce the number of calories that are going into your body. If you are still consuming more calories than your body is burning, you are still going to gain weight. It all goes back to the "calories consumed versus the calories burned" ratio. People are often amazed that they are able to still lose weight when they are eating larger portions of food that contains a lot of fat. All they are doing is taking away the calories that they would be consuming from carbohydrates and switching over to obtaining the calories from fat.

Another theory that has been out there for a while is that the more fat you eat, the less hungry you will be. That is a false statement and needs to be corrected. Your appetite gets suppressed when you are participating in a low-carbohydrate diet, because your body has gone into a state known as ketosis. When your body goes into that state, your appetite drops considerably, because your body's insulin levels have stabilized, and you no longer have to cope with unwanted cravings. If you were running out of food in the wild, you would not be able to handle the intensity of the hunger pangs that come along with not having food. In order for you to cope, your body switches from getting energy from the foods you eat over to utilizing the ketones that come from your stored body fat. When your body is utilizing the energy from its stored fat, it does not need additional nutrition, because it relies on stored energy. The element that I like most about being in a state of ketosis is that your cravings virtually disappear, and you are able to stick to the program much easier.

This program is quite easy once you are able to lock yourself into a state of ketosis. When you are in a state of ketosis, you will not be dealing with some of the same cravings that you have had in the past. If I feel as if I am beginning to get uncontrollable cravings, I always switch back to a low-carbohydrate diet until I feel I have that control back. One of the biggest drawbacks that low-carbohydrate dieting has is the scarceness of foods that you can eat, which is why I choose to eat a low-fat diet for maintenance, because my food choices are endless. The availability of food choices will not matter for this program, because the only thing we are concerned about here is getting results, and low-carbohydrate dieting is without question the most effective tool to get rid of the excess body fat.

One of the most important factors in any fat-loss program is the number of calories you consume. You already know that if you eat more calories than you consume, you are going to store fat, but what you may not know is how the body metabolizes energy. When you restrict calories in your diet, you end up lowering the amount of calories your body burns in a single day. When you withhold calories, your body sends a message to your metabolism to slow down so that you will be able to survive until more food is available. If you were ever in a situation that required you to go without food, you would fully appreciate this ability; however, when you are attempting to lose excess body fat, it can be one of the largest obstacles that you face.

One of the biggest obstacles I have had to deal with when it comes to dieting is being able to lose a lot of body fat and still keep the metabolic rate up. The reason yo-yo dieters always end up gaining more weight when they get off a diet is that they have altered the number of calories that their metabolism burns in a day. It is not uncommon to have your metabolism slow down by as much as 500 or more calories in a single day. For example, your body may currently be metabolizing 1,800 calories in a day. If you restrict the number of calories you consume to 1,000 calories in anticipation of burning 800 calories, your body will more than likely slow down to metabolizing 1,300 calories because of its need to conserve energy. That means that you are only burning approximately 300 calories in a single day. You will still lose weight over time, but any exercise you do will only be to compensate for the lowered number of calories your body is utilizing, which is why you will end up gaining the weight back when your diet is complete. You have to make sure that you maintain your metabolic rate throughout the entire diet.

The method that I utilize to keep your metabolism functioning at full capacity is to avoid dropping your caloric intake to less than 500 calories below the resting metabolic rate. You will learn more about your resting metabolic rate in the next section, but it is worth mentioning here, because the ability to manipulate your metabolism is one of the key elements that will ensure your success with this program.

When you are able to maintain a high metabolic rate and still lose a lot of fat, your body will be able to switch over to any diet plan you choose once you have lost all of the excess body fat, which is why the long-term results of this program far outweigh the quick fat loss that you will see in the mirror. I have been waiting for years for someone to put all of the pieces of the puzzle together in one program. It has been my experience that the majority of diet makers are more concerned with marketing their dieting concepts than they are with producing results. For some reason, they always leave out one the major components needed to ensure successful fat loss.

Many of the popular diets on the market today are catered toward a long-term lifestyle approach. The problem is, if you feel you are depriving yourself of something, you will eventually revert back to your prior eating habits. A diet should consist of fundamentals that give you results and also allow you to choose the foods you want to eat after you have lost all of the excess body fat. Maintaining your weight once you have lost all of the excess body fat will be much easier than you may think. I do not want you to get overloaded with all of the reasons I will be having you do some of the things you will be doing in this program, but I have to point out some of the biggest misconceptions about dieting.

Once you fully understand why I chose to structure this program the way that I have, you will be able to understand what is happening to your body at different stages of the program. With this program, you will be consuming enough calories to meet your daily caloric intake limit, but you will also be utilizing stored fat as your primary fuel source. When that happens, your body will end up burning stored body fat—even while you sleep! I hope that you are beginning to see why I have chosen to utilize the low-carbohydrate, controlled-calorie approach. It is the most aggressive form of burning stored body fat that is out there.

The problem that I have with the majority of the diets I have seen is that it is always their way or no way. If you are going to complete their diet, you have to make the adjustments for life. I have seen that approach fail time and time again. I do not know how anyone who could stick to a diet without understanding why they are doing it. Most people rely on the success of a friend to tell them how to lose weight, only to find that the friend gained all of that weight back a year later. Recognizing what is going on inside your body is one of the most important elements of any fat-loss program. Once you are provided with enough information, you will have no other choice but to consider what is going into your mouth.

When you are pigging out on a pizza, I am sure that you are not considering how many calories are going into your body, because if you did, you might not be able to eat it. One of the tools that I utilize in this program is giving you the freedom to choose how much you want to eat, as well as the freedom to choose when you want to eat. I utilize what I call the *banking system*. The banking system works by treating calories and carbohydrates as cash.

Every day, you will have a certain number of calories that you can spend any way you want to. Let's say that your resting metabolic rate is 1,800 calories. Every day, you will be able to consume up to 1,300 calories and up to 20 grams of carbohydrates. I do not care if you do not eat anything all day long and then, ten minutes before you go to bed, you eat all 1,300 calories. Your calories are for you to utilize in any way that you want to, just as long as you do not go over your limit. You will not be allowed to go over by even 10 calories.

When you are able to choose the foods that you like, you have the comfort of knowing that you can have whatever you want, as long as it does not go over your limits. The banking system is one of the simplest forms of maintaining a restricted-calorie diet. I utilize the banking system every day in my own life. Once you have been calculating your calories every day for a month, you will be able to start calculating the calories in your head. If I know that I am going to eat pizza in the evening, I know that I must restrict the number of calories that I consume earlier in the day.

When you are in the maintenance stage, you will be able to pay for extra consumed calories with exercise. That is even better, because when you really want to eat something that has a lot of calories, you just jump on the treadmill and pay for them. It is worth pointing out that when you get to that stage, you will be able to consume only what you have already paid for. If you want that extra piece of cake, you will have to pay for it first. Sorry, there are no loans made with this banking system. Why do you think credit-card companies make so much money? They know that it is easier to purchase something than it is to pay for it.

With this program, you will have a flexible food selection. I know that I will upset a lot of people in the health industry when I reveal that I tell clients that I do not care how many times they eat in a day. However, the truth of the matter is that it does not matter when you eat your meals, when it comes to fat loss, as long as you do not go over your limit. I agree that it is healthier for your body to absorb your meals over the course of a day, but when it comes to dieting, you are in control. The experts who state that it is healthier to break up your meals over a day are absolutely right. Smaller meals spread out throughout the day are better for your metabolism, because then your metabolism is always running. More nutrients will be absorbed by your body when you break them up over several meals.

I highly recommend that you do spread out your meals, but that decision is up to you. I know that in my busy life, I do not always have the time to eat every two hours. If you have a schedule that allows you to eat several meals throughout the day, great. But if you do not, you will still receive the results that come along with completing this program. I think that the banking system is probably one of the most flexible methods of controlling the number of calories and carbohydrates that you eat in a single day, which is why it is used in this program.

Once you are able to understand the benefits of the diet that I have chosen for this program, you will be able to prepare yourself for the types of foods that you will be able to eat in order to maintain a low-carbohydrate diet while still controlling the number of calories that are going into your body. I have dedicated an entire section of this program to informing you about the different foods you will be able to choose from.

Once you know what your selections will be, you will have a lot more flexibility with your diet. When you are eating out and the waiter advises you that the meal has only a certain amount of net carbohydrates, you need to realize that any form of carbohydrates in this program will count against your daily limit.

More and more food manufacturers have created substitutes for their products to lower the amount of carbohydrates that can be absorbed by the body. I think it is great that they are creating more options for the people who eat a low-carbohydrate diet, but none of these products are allowed in this program. I have seen too many of my clients stagnate in their fat-loss efforts by adding these products to their diet. If you want to maintain a low-carbohydrate lifestyle, I do not see a problem with these products. But while you are in this program, you have to count every carbohydrate as a carbohydrate, whether it can be absorbed by the body or not.

It may be difficult for you to resist the temptation to eat something that indicates it only has a certain amount of net carbohydrates, but I assure you that it will affect the results you receive from this program. I cannot tell you how many times some of my clients have obtained their food sources from products that represented only a certain amount of "impact carbohydrates," but they were never able to lose as much fat as my clients who adhered to my stricter carbohydrate rules. There is a mental factor that comes into play when you feel that you are eating too many carbohydrates. If you believe that you are cheating yourself, you will be much more tempted to quit the program. You will definitely be overstepping your boundaries if you attempt to trick yourself into believing that you are only getting a certain amount of carbohydrates from a meal, as in an instance of a label that states a meal has fifty grams of carbohydrates but only three of those grams count. I have a major problem with the mental suggestion that labels such as those give you.

Another thing that I want you to avoid consuming for the entire program is carbonated beverages. If you like diet sodas, you will be able to drink as many as you like once you're off this program, but I have had too many clients stagnate in their fat-loss results by drinking soda. Once you are able to clear your system of the mess that carbonation was creating, you will experience the benefits of drinking non-carbonated beverages. A diet soda usually does not have any carbohydrates in it, so you may be very tempted to add this to your diet.

You have to understand that your body will be breaking down a significant amount of stored body fat over the next thirty days. You have to aid it any way you can. When you ask your body to secrete fat through your pores via carbonation, you're asking for toxicity. Please listen to this warning—I would not have made it a requirement if it weren't absolutely necessary. The only beverages you should be consuming are water and other pure forms of hydration that have the least amount of ingredients in it. You will never go wrong with water, so I suggest that you consider making water your only form of hydration for the next thirty days.

I believe that you are beginning to see the shape of the entire program. The main principle is to stay within your boundaries, and when you do that, you will be able to complete this program without any interruptions. The moment you decide to step outside of those boundaries, you are going to fail, and you will have to begin the program over from scratch. It has been my experience that the people who successfully complete this program are the ones who stay within their boundaries from the beginning. Every time you fail on this program, it will become more difficult to succeed, so get ready! Educate yourself about why you are doing this program, and enjoy the results.

In the next section, we will be discussing how to determine the number of calories you will be able to consume in a day. I hope you have a better understanding of why I have chosen the diet that I have, because the more information you are provided with, the greater chance you will have of completing this program.

Calculating Caloric Intake Limit

Before you will be able to determine your daily caloric-intake limit, you will have to formulate your resting metabolic rate. The resting metabolic rate is also known as the basal rate. The basal rate is the number of calories your body burns in a twenty-four-hour period when your body is at complete rest. If you are bedridden or you live a very sedentary lifestyle, the basal rate is utilized to determine the number of calories you need in order to maintain your current weight. If you are active and exercise regularly, you will be able to factor in the number of calories you burn during these activities. This will create a more accurate calculation of the number of calories you should be consuming in order to maintain your current weight.

This program will not be factoring in the additional number of calories you will burn during exercise. I am only concerned with your resting metabolic rate, because this is the magic number we will be utilizing to maximize fat loss and keep your metabolism burning more calories than you are consuming, without decreasing its efficiency. When you limit your caloric intake to 500 calories below your basal rate, you will experience the most effective way to keep your metabolism working at full capacity.

The equation we are going to utilize to determine your basal rate is called the Harris-Benedict Equation. This equation is the most effective method for determining your basal rate from a calculation. It is also the most common equation that physicians and dietitians use. In order to determine your basal rate, you first need to convert your body weight from pounds into kilograms, which is achieved when you take your weight in pounds and divide it by 2.204.

For example, if you weigh 200 pounds, you should divide 200 by 2.204, which equals 90.74. When you round that number up, you get 91 kilograms. Once you have your weight in kilograms, you need to convert your height from inches into centimeters, which is accomplished by multiplying 2.54 by your height in inches. For example, if you are 6 feet tall, you should multiply 72 inches by 2.54, which equals 182.88. When you round that number up, you get 183 centimeters. Now that you have your weight in kilograms and your height in centimeters, you are ready to calculate your basal rate from the following equation.

Men: 66.5 + (13.75 X kg) + (5.003 X cm) – (6.775 X age)
Women: 655.1 + (9.563 X kg) + (1.850 X cm) – (4.676 X age)

If you are a 50-year-old man, weighing 200 pounds and 6 feet tall, your resting metabolic rate is 1,895.

If you are a 50-year-old woman, weighing 200 pounds and 6 feet tall, your resting metabolic rate is 1,630.

Now that you have established your resting metabolic rate, you will need to subtract 500 from that number, and you will have your daily caloric-intake limit. Now that you have the magic number that you will not be able to go over, we need to establish the parameters that go along with restricting your daily caloric intake.

Under no circumstance will you be allowed to go over your daily caloric-intake limit. If your resting metabolic rate is 1,800, your daily limit will be set at 1,300. Please keep in mind that not every product that you purchase will have the correct nutritional content on the label, so you will have to give yourself a cushion to allow for mistakes. When you go over your limit even by 10 calories, it will have an impact on your results and hence on your confidence.

I need to point out why I use only your resting metabolic rate without factoring in the extra calories you will burn during exercise: because the calories you burn during exercise will come directly from your stored body fat. The more calories you can remove from your body, the more body fat you will lose. If you factor in the calories you burn during exercise, you would never get ahead. When you switch back to a more flexible way of eating, you will appreciate the ability to burn the same, if not more, calories than you did prior to losing the excess body fat. Not only are you maintaining your metabolic rate, but you will weigh less and still burn the same number of calories as when you were heavier.

Over the next thirty days, your body will be transformed into a highly tuned fat-burning machine. This has always been my specialty, and I hope that you stay committed long enough to enjoy it. When your body is burning fat, even while you sleep, you are going to lose more body fat then you could possibly imagine. Your metabolism believes that it is getting all of the calories that it needs, so it does not slow down; however, you are not fueling it with carbohydrates, so you are directly burning stored fat. It is a powerful trick of manipulation, but your body will appreciate the results it obtains from it.

I have just shown you one of the most powerful tools in the personal training business. I have transformed many lives by using this very simple procedure. The problem with low-fat diets is that they rely on exercise in order to lose the fat, and the problem with low-carbohydrate diets is that they do not control the number of calories that an individual can consume while dieting. The secret is to combine both of the most effective elements into one diet. When you do that, you have the ability to burn fat even while you are sleeping!

Now that you have been able to formulate your own personal magic number, you are ready to put your body in a state of ketosis! When your body is in a state of ketosis, you will not only be burning a lot of fat, but you will have control over your hunger for possibly the first time in your life. Determining your daily caloric-intake limit was the first step in setting your parameters. Now it is time to discuss putting your body into ketosis. This process will be discussed in its entirety in the following section.

Entering Ketosis

Ketosis is achieved by reducing the amount of carbohydrates that you consume to a level low enough to make your body utilize incompletely metabolized fats (ketone bodies) for energy. When you enter a state of ketosis, you are increasing the amount of ketone bodies present within your body. This means that you are releasing stored fat from your body and secreting it through your breath and digestive system.

The more ketones that are in your urine, the deeper into a state of ketosis you may be in. However, an increase in ketone bodies could also mean that you are not consuming enough water. In this program, you will not be permitted to consume more than twenty grams of carbohydrates in a single day. By restricting carbs in this way, you put your body into a forced state of ketosis.

Then, when you exercise, you utilize the stored fat in your body for energy. You also utilize the stored fat in your body while you sleep. As you learned in the previous section, your body burns a certain number of calories, even when you are not active, which is why you will even burn fat as you sleep! Your body will be literally breaking down fat and utilizing it for energy at all hours of the day.

When you consume more carbohydrates in your diet, your body utilizes those carbohydrates for fuel before it utilizes stored fat. When you are consuming higher levels of carbohydrates, you may burn stored fat only when you exercise for prolonged periods of time. When you are in a state of ketosis, exercise is a bonus. Exercising while you are in a state of ketosis is what produces the intense results that make this program so effective.

There are a lot of misconceptions about the safety of being in ketosis, which is primarily attributable to the lack of research regarding the effects of prolonged periods of ketosis. One of the biggest misconceptions is that individuals in a state of ketosis suffer from the same symptoms as individuals who have Type I diabetes. This is simply not true. Type I diabetics are victims of a pathological condition that lowers the body's amount of insulin and hinders the body's ability to restrain adrenaline, noradrenaline, and glucagons. When this happens, the body burns excessive amounts of fat, which can cause a deterioration of bodily tissue. When you are in a voluntary state of dietary-induced ketosis, your body is burning only the stored fat that it has available. If you were to continue to restrict your calories once you lost the majority of your body fat, you would eventually start burning away healthy muscle. If you decide to stay on a low-carbohydrate diet once you have lost all of the excess body fat, you will need to elevate the number of calories you consume in order to preserve the muscle that is fueling your metabolism.

Another popular misconception is that ketosis is a toxic state. That is an old belief that has been corrected by several clinical studies. Researchers were first concerned that the ketone bodies were toxic-waste products, because they felt that the brain could not properly function when it was forced to utilize ketones as energy. In a series of studies conducted in 1967, researchers discovered that the human brain was able to utilize ketone bodies for fuel during prolonged periods of starvation. This changed the entire outlook on ketosis for physicians and dietitians. In more recent news, ketogenic (low-carb) diets have gained an amazingly large amount of publicity because of the vast number of health benefits that come along with low-carbohydrate dieting. It is difficult to enter a grocery store without locating a section that is dedicated to low-carbohydrate diets. The majority of fast-food restaurants have added low-carbohydrate alternatives as well.

One of the main reasons I chose to use a ketogenic diet for this program is that it is the most aggressive way to safely lose stored body fat. However, there is another very important factor that comes along with being in the state of ketosis. This factor is without question one of the most effective tools for ridding your body of excess fat. This wonderful tool is *appetite suppression*. When you no longer have hunger pangs and you no longer feel the need to eat all the time, you have a lot more control of your diet.

It takes approximately forty-eight hours to enter ketosis once you reduce carbohydrates to less than twenty grams per day. You can speed up this process by exercising. I am not going to have you exercise to speed this process up, because when your body switches from utilizing from carbohydrates for energy and converts over to utilizing ketone bodies, you may experience some temporary side effects. That is why it is always important to stay under the close supervision of your physician. Some of the possible side effects may include nausea, diarrhea, fatigue, and irritability. These side effects may sound bad, but it is worth pointing out that though they may happen as you start to enter into ketosis, once you have safely gotten your body converted over to burning ketone bodies, any side effects that you may experience will probably disappear. Most people give up before their bodies have gotten a chance to completely make the conversion. As a result, they never get the opportunity to experience the benefits that go along with being in ketosis.

Once you start the program, I will give you a lot of guidance each day so that you will not be alarmed at what is going on with your body. This will help reassure you that everything will be OK once you have successfully converted over to burning ketone bodies for fuel.

When your body stores excess body fat, it is because you are consuming more calories than what is required to complete your daily activities. If you eat 2,000 calories in a single day, you have to burn off that many calories in order not to store energy. The math is extremely simple, but it requires conscious thought to keep track of it. This program works like a vacuum cleaner. Yes, it will be sucking up the mess you made, but it will be your responsibility to maintain the results.

When your body is not held down by all the excess body fat, you are going to have an abundance of energy. You already know that your body does not like the methods you are currently utilizing to maintain it, so it is time to change. By entering ketosis, you will be taking one of the most important steps toward relieving your body of excess body fat. After you have depleted your body of all that extra fat, it will be free to operate at full capacity. You cannot overlook the importance of taking care of yourself; just keep in mind that any minor discomfort that you may experience as you enter ketosis is only temporary. The results you achieve will last a lifetime.

One of the elements that I have included in this program is ketone-testing strips. You can purchase these testing strips at any local pharmacy. Most testing strips provide four or more colors to indicate the varying levels of ketones that are present in your urine. I have seen testing strips on the market that had only two color indicators, and that will not suffice for this program. The most common strips start with a light pink color and work their way up to a dark purple color. These strips will be the primary tool utilized throughout this program to ensure that you are maintaining your state of ketosis.

On the day you start this program, you will probably not indicate even a trace amount of ketones, but by the third day, your ketone-testing strip should be indicating a moderate to large amount of ketones in your system. If you are not registering even a trace amount of ketones by the third day, you will know that you are consuming too many carbohydrates. These strips do not lie, and because I do not want you measuring yourself until after the program is complete, they will be the main motivating factor to let you know that you are burning stored fat as energy.

You will need to make sure that you hold your testing strip in your stream of urine for just a second. If you hold it under the stream for too long, it may rinse off some of the chemicals used to measure the amount of ketones in your urine. You may also choose to urinate into a cup and dip the testing strip into the cup to ensure that you are not rinsing the chemicals off. You will be required to test for ketones every morning. I have found that the first urination of the day always yields the most accurate results.

Once you are indicating a large amount of ketones on your testing strip, you will be required to maintain that amount throughout the entire program. You will want to purchase these testing strips before you start the first day of the program. Even though it may take you a few days to enter ketosis, I want you to see how long it takes your body to go into this state. It will serve as a reminder of how long it takes for your body to use up all the stored carbohydrates in your system. Once you get into the habit of testing for ketones, you will actually start to look forward to obtaining that validation every day. It is a visible reminder of the amount of fat your body is removing every day.

Food Selection

In order to conveniently plan your diet, you will need to have a good idea as to what types of food you will be permitted to eat. When you are restricted to only twenty grams of carbohydrates in a day, you are going to have to plan out your daily diet in advance. If you were on a typical low-carbohydrate diet, they would tell you to eat as much food as you wanted, as long as you did not go over your limit of carbohydrates. With this program, this is not the case. We will restrict the number of calories that are going into your body as well. When you restrict the number of calories that are going into your body, you will have to be even more cautious about the foods that you consume.

Many foods that are low in carbohydrates are also very high in fat. The convenient feature for you is that you can spend your calories any way you wish. If you want something that is higher in fat, all you have to do is cut back the total volume of food you consume for that day. When you are in ketosis, you are going to have a lot more flexibility, because you will have control over your appetite. Staying below your maximum caloric and carbohydrate limit will not be difficult once you can control your hunger.

I am going to list some of the most common foods that you will have to choose from and provide their caloric and carbohydrate totals. Some of the items I have listed are not going to be permitted in your diet; I just wanted you to see how high they are in carbohydrates. If you do not know the nutritional content of a food that you are considering eating, do not eat it. You need to always pay attention to what is put into your food. You may be at a restaurant and feel safe ordering a chicken breast. But what did they put on that chicken breast? You have to be almost obsessive about the number of calories and carbohydrates that you consume for the next thirty days. At the end of this program, you will be able to calculate the numbers in your head, but while you are in this program, you will have to keep precise track of your total intake every day.

Now that you know your caloric intake limit and that you cannot go over twenty grams of carbohydrates in a single day, you are ready to go to the grocery store and get your fat-burning foods! I hope this will help you have a better idea of the foods to consume and the foods to avoid. You will possibly notice that there are several food groups that I left out of this section. I chose to do this because it is obvious that bread, fruit, pasta, and sweets are high in carbohydrates and cannot even be considered until after you have completed this program. The nutrient totals below are not always exact—you will still need to look at the nutritional content on the labels of the foods you choose to include into your diet.

Meat, Poultry, Shellfish:

Chicken breast (1 pound with bone)	0.0 carbohydrates	390	calories
Ground beef (1 pound lean)	0.0 carbohydrates	815	calories
Ham (1 pound with bone and skin)	0.0 carbohydrates	1,190	calories
Shrimp (1 pound with shell)	5.0 carbohydrates	290	calories
Sirloin steak (1 pound with bone)	0.0 carbohydrates	1,240	calories

Vegetables:

Asparagus (1 pound untrimmed)	13.0 carbohydrates	65	calories
Avocado (10.7 ounces, 1 fruit)	14.5 carbohydrates	250	calories
Broccoli (1 pound untrimmed)	16.5 carbohydrates	70	calories
Celery (1 pound untrimmed)	13.5 carbohydrates	60	calories
Cucumber (8 ounces with peel)	7.5 carbohydrates	30	calories
Green beans (1 pound untrimmed)	28.5 carbohydrates	130	calories
Lettuce (1 pound iceberg)	1.5 carbohydrates	60	calories
Mushroom (1 pound untrimmed)	19.5 carbohydrates	120	calories
Okra (1 pound untrimmed)	29.5 carbohydrates	140	calories
Onion (1 pound untrimmed)	36.0 carbohydrates	155	calories
Summer squash (1 pound)	19.0 carbohydrates	90	calories
Tomato (1 pound untrimmed)	21.5 carbohydrates	100	calories
White cabbage (1 pound)	19.5 carbohydrates	90	calories

Dairy:

Cheese (1 ounce American/cheddar)	0.5 carbohydrates	105	calories
Cheese (1 ounce Colby)	1.0 carbohydrates	110	calories

Cheese (1 ounce mozzarella)	0.0 carbohydrates	80	calories
Cheese (1 ounce Parmesan)	1.0 carbohydrates	110	calories
Cheese (4 ounces cottage)	4.0 carbohydrates	110	calories
Milk (8 ounces skim)	12.0 carbohydrates	90	calories
Sour cream (1 tablespoon)	1.0 carbohydrates	25	calories
Yogurt (8 ounces plain nonfat)	18.0 carbohydrates	130	calories

Condiments:

Barbecue sauce (1 tablespoon)	3.0 carbohydrates	15	calories
Fresh herbs (1 tablespoon)	0.5 carbohydrates	10	calories
Ketchup (1 teaspoon)	4.0 carbohydrates	15	calories
Mayonnaise (1 teaspoon)	0.0 carbohydrates	100	calories
Mustard (1 teaspoon)	0.5 carbohydrates	5	calories
Salsa (1 teaspoon)	1.0 carbohydrates	5	calories
Soy sauce (1 ounce)	3.0 carbohydrates	20	calories
Tabasco sauce (1 teaspoon)	0.0 carbohydrates	0	calories
Tartar sauce (1 teaspoon)	0.5 carbohydrates	75	calories
Teriyaki sauce (1 teaspoon)	3.0 carbohydrates	15	calories
Worcestershire sauce (1 teaspoon)	3.0 carbohydrates	10	calories

Nutritional Supplementation

I cannot stress enough the importance of including multivitamins in your daily life. You must take multivitamins to participate in this program. I would like to clear up a lot of the confusion about multivitamins. You have possibly heard someone say that they are nothing more than expensive urine, but I disagree, and so do the majority of physicians. On any given day, are you going to eat all of the foods needed in order to maintain your nutritional needs? More than likely, you will not. It is very difficult to know if your body is getting the vitamins and minerals that it needs in order to properly function.

When you participate in a program of this nature, you will have to supplement your diet with the vitamins that you are missing out on. You may have seen low-carbohydrate diets that recommend eating more vegetables, and they are partially correct, but you must keep in mind that vegetables contain carbohydrates. When you eat a salad, you have to make certain that you do not underestimate the amount of carbohydrates that are in the vegetables. When you are limiting your carbohydrate intake to less than twenty grams per day, you are going to have to supplement your diet with a multivitamin. A multivitamin will not only maintain your health but will also aid in the fat-burning process taking place within your body.

One of the factors to consider is the type of multivitamin to take. I am going to list each vitamin separately and show you the function it performs within your body. Once you know what vitamins you need, I'll discuss the dosage of each vitamin that you need to take. Once you have determined the proper vitamins and the proper dosages to ingest, you will be able to maintain a healthy level of the essential vitamins and minerals that your body will need to get you through this program. I always recommend taking a vitamin immediately following a meal. Studies have shown that this greatly increases the chance of the vitamin getting absorbed into your body. I also recommend getting a higher-strength vitamin, in which the dosage can be divided throughout the day, which will also increase the chances of getting more of the vitamins and minerals into your body.

The vitamins that I recommend you take are listed below. I hope you will gain a better understanding of why you need to supplement your diet with a really powerful multivitamin.

Vitamin A (Beta Carotene/Acetate)
Recommended daily intake: 10,000 IU
Bodily function: vision, bone growth, glands, hair
Sources: dairy products, green and yellow vegetables

Vitamin C (Calcium Ascorbate)
Recommended daily intake: 360 mg
Bodily function: immune system, bone and tooth formation, iron absorption
Sources: citrus fruits, green vegetables, horseradish, tomatoes, strawberries

Vitamin D (Cholecalciferol)
Recommended daily intake: 400 mg
Bodily function: bones, cartilage, heart, nervous system, collagen
Sources: milk, tuna, egg yolks, natural sunlight

Vitamin E (d-Alpha Tocopheryl)
Recommended daily intake: 400 IU
Bodily function: skin, muscle metabolism, heart, collagen
Sources: green vegetables, nuts, seeds, cabbage, yeast

Vitamin K (Phytonadione)
Recommended daily intake: 80 mcg
Bodily function: blood circulation, growth
Sources: soy beans, potatoes, eggs, tomatoes

Vitamin B-1 (Thiamin)
Recommended daily intake: 25 mg
Bodily function: growth, digestion, muscle, metabolism, energy
Sources: green vegetables, nuts, raisins, potatoes, corn

Vitamin B-2 (Riboflavin)
Recommended daily intake: 25 mg
Bodily function: vision, skin, hair
Sources: green vegetables, liver, cheese, avocados, milk, nuts

Vitamin B-3 (Niacin)
Recommended daily intake: 20 mcg
Bodily function: metabolism, digestive system, fat synthesis
Sources: liver, fish, poultry, beef, avocados, potatoes, cheese

Vitamin B-5 (Pantotothenic Acid)
Recommended daily intake: 60 mg
Bodily function: metabolism, skin, digestion
Sources: liver, fish, poultry, beef, avocados, eggs, nuts

Vitamin B-6 (Pyridoxine HCI)
Recommended daily intake: 25 mg
Bodily function: metabolism, red blood cells, nerve tissue
Sources: liver, fish, beef, poultry, green vegetables

Vitamin B-12 (Cyanocobalamin)
Recommended daily intake: 200 mcg
Bodily function: metabolism, memory, cell production
Sources: liver, beef, eggs, shellfish

Folic Acid
Recommended daily intake: 600 mcg
Bodily function: metabolism, hair, red blood cells
Sources: green vegetables, liver, nuts, grains

Biotin
Recommended daily intake: 300 mcg
Bodily function: metabolism, skin, hair, bone marrow
Sources: beef, liver, eggs, soybeans, milk

Calcium (Phosphate/Citrate/Ascorbate)
Recommended daily intake: 300 mg
Bodily function: bone formation, blood clotting, muscle
Source: milk, green vegetables, beans, shellfish

Magnesium
Recommended daily intake: 400 mg
Bodily function: energy, bones, muscles, nerves
Source: green vegetables, meat, beans, milk, eggs

Zinc (Monomethionine)
Recommended daily intake: 20 mg
Bodily function: immune system, blood, insulin, cell growth
Source: shellfish, green vegetables, poultry, eggs, nuts

Selenium (Sodium Selenate)
Recommended daily intake: 75 mcg
Bodily function: metabolism
Sources: meat, shellfish, green vegetables, onions, tomatoes

Copper
Recommended daily intake: 2 mcg
Bodily function: bone growth, skin, collagen
Sources: shellfish, liver, nuts

Manganese
Recommended daily intake: 1 mg
Bodily function: metabolism
Sources: green vegetables, beans, eggs, liver

Chromium
Recommended daily intake: 300 mcg
Bodily function: metabolism, energy, insulin
Sources: meat, cheese, corn oil

Now that you have a list of the vitamins and minerals that I have selected, it is time to go to the store and purchase them. You can take this program with you if you need to compare the contents. The vitamins and dosages I have selected cater to a low-carbohydrate diet. The dosages on some of the vitamin containers may be difficult to locate, but do the best that you can. Any multivitamin is better than no multivitamin.

PART III
Exercise

Exercise Fundamentals

Now that you have established the self-discipline that you will need to complete this program, you have calculated your caloric-intake limit, and you understand why you must stay under twenty grams of carbohydrates a day, you are ready for the last element in the Intense Trainer Program. Without exercise, you will not be able to obtain intense results. The reason I have built such a strong foundation is that it will take strength in order to handle the exercise portion of this program. I am going to utilize a cardiovascular exercise in your daily routine.

In order for you to fully appreciate how beneficial exercising is for your body, we need to discuss what will be taking place while you are working out. If you are consuming 1,800 calories in a single day, you already know that you need to burn 1,800 calories in order to not gain weight. You know that you will have to burn more calories than you are consuming in order to get the intense results that you are seeking.

I have you stay 500 calories under your resting metabolic rate because I want to fully utilize your body's stored fat as energy. The reason you are allowed to consume up to your daily caloric-intake limit is that I do not want to lower your metabolic rate. If you go under your resting metabolic rate by more than 500 calories, your metabolism will sense that you are withholding food, and it will automatically slow down. We cannot afford to have that rate slow down. The moment we add exercise into your program, I want your metabolism to be working at full capacity.

In fact, I am going to assist you in raising that metabolic rate higher than what it was when you had all the excess body fat. That is the trick to getting your body to burn as many calories as it can in a single day. By the time you start your program, you will have already established your discipline and dieting needs. All that will be left are the intense workouts. This is the part you have been getting ready for. I am going to absolutely push your body to the maximum each and every day.

This section of the program will enable you to shed massive amounts of fat in a very short period of time. If your foundation had not been poured, you would not be able to complete this section of the program.

In order for you to be able to say that you successfully completed the Intense Trainer Program, you will not be allowed to skip one step. I will discuss that later in the program, but it is worth mentioning here, because I expect you to complete this program in its entirety, which includes finishing the exercises that I designed for you. You will not be permitted to skip even one minute of exercise.

The importance of exercising will speak for itself when you see your body transform before your eyes. This experience will possibly be one of the most invigorating experiences of your life. Finishing a program, knowing that you did not skip one step, and forcing yourself to abide by the parameters that you have set will not only boost your level of self-esteem, it will change your entire life. You will be able to accomplish anything you set your mind to, because you will have both mental energy and physical energy.

We have already discussed the role of mental energy, so it is now time to discuss the importance of physical energy. When you exercise, you are obviously burning energy, but did you know that you are training your body to create more energy? When you actively train your body to withstand the increasing demands that you are placing on it, you are actually training your body to utilize energy more efficiently.

As you learned in the dieting section of this program, your metabolism can only burn what your body expends. Energy is no different. Energy is created by the requirements of your body. If all you do in a day is sit on your couch in the living room and watch television, your body's energy level is going to adjust to that. If you are jogging for thirty minutes a day, your body is going to have to adjust to that need as well. You really need to pay close attention to this, because this very powerful tool will get you through this program. Think about it: why is it that the more energy you expend, the more energy you have? If you go for a thirty-minute jog at night, why is it so hard to sleep afterward? The answer to this question is the reason why you have to increase the energy demands that you place on your body.

Your body is only doing what you tell it to do. The body was designed to maximize your enjoyment in life. If you tell your body that all you want to do is sit on the couch, it will do what it needs to in order to accommodate you. Your body's image is a direct reflection of what you are telling it you want to do. When I see someone who is overweight, I know that they have not been expecting much out of their body.

The body's energy level can make or break any diet plan, especially one like this. You have to start asking more out of your body than what is required to just get you through the day. Once you start to feel the benefits that come along with exercising, you will no longer look at it as work. You will start to create something of an addiction to it. It may be the healthiest addiction you have ever had, but it is an addiction nonetheless.

Once you have the energy to work out, you will need to know what kind of exercises to do. One of the most effective exercises for burning fat is jogging. If you are fortunate enough to have a treadmill, you will be able to take full advantage of it now. I have utilized many different forms of machinery in and out of the gym, but none have been able to take off fat more quickly than jogging. If you are really out of shape, I am going to discuss the methods you will need to follow in order to be able to jog for an extended period of time. Jogging, like every other form of exercise, requires exertion. You have to start out slow and build your way up. If you are older or are carrying a substantial amount of weight on your body, I am going to discuss what kind of walking you should start out with.

When it comes to exercising, people appear to have a lot of excuses why they cannot do it. I have created the ultimate solution to all of these somewhat complex excuses. I have spent a lot of time studying the most common reasons why someone does not work out. I have been able to narrow down all of the secondary reasons into one main reason. The main reason why people do not exercise is time management. Poor time management is the most destructive excuse that I have had to deal with. It is always easy to work out when you have plenty of spare time, but it is a different story when your daily agenda starts to swell, and you seem to always have to squeeze in time for exercising.

We have to remedy that problem before it gets out of control. In order to maintain control of your exercise schedule, we have to create a plan that will eliminate worries about missing a workout. This solution is one that my own mind fought me on for years. It would be an understatement to say that I am not exactly a morning person. I have always preferred to work out at night, because I have always been a night owl. My body does not even want to function until after 10 AM.

My clients are the ones who changed my outlook on morning workouts. For years, I spent the majority of my time working late into the evening, so it was natural for me to want to sleep in. This all changed when I had to be waiting at a health club at 5 AM for my first client. If you are going to make it as a personal trainer, you are going to have to always be fully charged for every workout that you administer. My clients expect all of me every time they train with me. If I am having an off day, they will sense it, and the workout will falter as a result of it.

When I had to begin waking up at 4 AM in order to have time to cook breakfast, take a shower, and feed the dog, I was pushing it to arrive by 5 AM. Then, other factors started to play into my schedule. At one point, I had thirty full-time clients. A full-time client is any individual who trains with me a minimum of twice a week, which translates into more than sixty hours a week that I trained on the floor with my clients. If you have not had the opportunity to train with me in person, it may be somewhat difficult to fully understand the intensity of my workouts. They are equally tough on me as they are on the clients who I am training. I often have to shower several times a day as a result of the amount of effort I put into training a client.

If a client was having difficulty with a jogging routine, I would occasionally jog with him or her for free, just to understand why he or she was struggling. This could translate into more than fifteen miles a day that I would spend jogging with clients. Even though I spent many hours participating in cardiovascular exercises with my clients, I still had to complete my own strength-training exercises at the end of the day. By the end of the day, I did not have enough time to complete my own routine. I would spend twelve hours a day in a gym and still not get my own workout completed.

I knew at that point that I had to change my schedule in order to ensure that I would get my own quality workout in. In order for me to do this, I was forced, and I do mean forced, to work out at 3 AM. I never thought in a million years that I would have to wake up at 3 AM to complete my own workout, but I did. The only way that you will ever be able to ensure that you will complete your daily workout is to do it first thing in the morning. Feeling that you will not be able to because you will not get enough sleep is just another excuse for not adjusting your daily schedule.

I hate to say it, but it's worth repeating: the only way you can consistently ensure that you will obtain your daily workout is to do it first thing in the morning. I assure you, there is no one who would more strongly prefer this was not the case than me, but it is necessary to ensure that you continue not only to lose body fat but also to maintain the results that you receive.

The upside to working out first thing in the morning is the massive amount of energy that you start your day with. Over time, my body has learned that it actually requires this energy in order to keep up with the busy schedule that I have. Some people require a cup of coffee to get them moving in the morning, but I grab a dumbbell instead. I am certain that my habit is healthier for my body than a cup of coffee would be—what do you think?

The ability to manage your daily activities is a direct result of your level of discipline. I am going to have you work out first thing in the morning because it is going to take all you have just to complete this program. I am not going to add another excuse to your growing list of reasons why you cannot work out. Instead, you will know if you are going to fail this program within the first hour after you wake up. You will not have to wonder whether you will successfully complete your daily schedule, because you will have already accomplished the most difficult portion of the program.

Now that we have addressed the main excuse, "I don't have enough time," it is time to look at a lot of the secondary excuses, which all lead back to time management. The second most common excuse that I hear is "I was so stressed out that I didn't get a chance to work out." We know that time management can eliminate this excuse, but there is another common excuse that I hear a lot, even from the clients who were working out first thing in the morning: "I didn't have enough energy."

I have discussed the importance of building up your energy level early in this section, but I am going to provide you with a more direct look at what it takes to create this newly discovered energy. We, as humans, are creatures of habit. What we consistently expend is what we will consistently receive in return. When you train your body to withstand thirty minutes of cardiovascular exercising, you are not training your body as much as you're training your mind. Your body will get on the treadmill, but your mind will want to fight you.

I never want to hear you say that you cannot do something in this program. If you are a healthy individual, there will be nothing in this program that you cannot do if you take the time to mentally prepare for it. If you are this far into the program and you have not been able to understand the importance of disciplining yourself to support your beliefs, you need to start over, slow down, and really take the time to fully understand how self-discipline works. Everything in this program leads back to discipline, so if you skipped that section, you are not going to be able to move on until you have a clear understanding as to why you need it.

When you say that you will do something, you are assuming control over your body's motor responses. If you say that you're going to walk across the floor, your body is going to do what it needs to in order to accommodate your request. If you say that you will walk on the treadmill, your body is going to accommodate you.

In the next section, I will discuss what I am going to do for you if you are not currently in good shape. Your success in jogging is reliant on your body's ability to do it. If you are a healthy individual, you should at least be able to start out at a fast walk and build your way up to a thirty-minute jog. When clients tell me that they do not have enough energy to at least walk for thirty minutes, I immediately have to address their false and limiting beliefs, because that is just what they are—false and limiting beliefs.

Another reason people have so much difficulty exercising is that they do not maintain their mental self-discipline long enough to make their bodies consistently do it. The ability to exercise seven days a week comes from the ability to do it long enough to create a new habit. Good habits take time to establish, just as bad habits do. Once you have been working out consistently for thirty days, your body is going to be able to do anything that you want it to do. The problem is that most people get consumed by their own negative thoughts, and they never get a chance to discover the pleasant joy that comes along with exercising.

When your body gets into the habit of pushing healthy oxygen through your cardiovascular system, you will start to feel the need to do it every day. If I am out of town on business, I will jog in place if I have to. My body has gotten into the habit of working out, so it has to have exercise in order to feel good.

Up until now, you have probably created the types of habits that are unconsciously destructive to the things that you want in life. There is a reason you picked up this program. I went out of my way to discourage the weaker portion of the public from purchasing this program. I saved this program for the individuals, like you, who know that they have what it takes to have anything they want in life. Think about it: out of all of the programs out there that you could have chosen from, you chose the most intense one of them all. Why is that? There has to be a reason that you feel that you have what it takes to push yourself to the absolute limit. I congratulate you for making it this far, assuming that you have read the entire program up to this point.

You must keep in mind that you do not want to start this program if you are still not certain about the need to have self-discipline. I hope that you are the type of person who will stick to at least one thing in your life for at least thirty short days. Every day that you complete your morning exercise is a day that you will be able to say you accomplished something that most people can only dream about.

Most people are so consumed with worrying how hard something seems that they never get to experience how easy that thing can be when it does not feel like work. But this program will change your entire outlook on exercising. If you think that it is going to be work, it will be; however, if you stay with it long enough, you won't know how you ever lived without it. The ability to exercise seven days a week is created by making sure that you do it before you start your day. Once you start your day with an accomplishment, imagine how well the rest of your day will go!

Cardiovascular Training

Cardiovascular exercises are the backbone of the Intense Trainer Program. This one element is, without question, the most effective tool I will utilize to shed stored fat from your body. I cannot stress enough how important it is for you not to miss even one scheduled cardiovascular workout session. I need to remind you that this program is designed to last for only thirty days. At the end of that thirty-day time span, you will have developed all of the necessary habits to ensure a lifetime of health and fitness. In order to back that claim up, I will need you to complete the entire program, which includes every cardiovascular workout session. Before you are able to fully understand the importance of cardiovascular exercise, you need to know what your body is actually doing as you work out. Once you have gained a better understanding of what your body is doing, you will understand why cardiovascular exercise is one of the requirements of this program.

Cardiovascular training enhances the lungs' ability to exchange oxygen and carbon dioxide in the blood, and it assists the circulatory system's ability to transport blood and nutrients to your body's metabolically active tissues for sustained periods of time without causing unnecessary fatigue. You will train your body to circulate greater amounts of oxygen and nutrients so that you are able to jog for longer periods of time.

When your body is functioning with a highly conditioned circulatory system, you will be able to accomplish more of the things that you want to do in life. If you want to lose body fat, you have to exercise. In order to be able to exercise, you will need a body that is not going to fatigue after the first couple of minutes. Too many people fail an exercise program before they get a chance to properly train their cardiovascular system. The stronger your cardiovascular system becomes, the more exercise you will be able to do, and with less effort.

Some people are able to run every day, because they have properly trained their bodies to be able to run for extended periods of time. Once your body is able to exercise for greater periods of time, you will be able to burn more calories with less effort. The more oxygen you have pumping through your body, the healthier you will feel. If you have ever had the opportunity to run for extended periods of time, you may have already experienced what is called *runner's high*.

This feeling of being high is a result of the increased amount of oxygen circulating through your system. This euphoric feeling makes you feel as if you could literally run for hours. I hope that you will experience this amazing sensation before the end of this program. As your cardiovascular system improves, you have the opportunity to increase the intensity of your workouts. When you start to do that, you will know that you are heading in the right direction.

I have discussed some of the ways cardiovascular training assists your body in losing excess body fat, but it's also important to point out some of the health benefits that go along with cardiovascular training. Some of the most common health benefits are: a reduction in blood pressure; decreased levels of cholesterol; decreased storing of body fat; decreased symptoms of depression, anxiety, and tension; increased heart function; decreased chances of dying after a heart attack; decreased chances of developing Type II diabetes; increased ability to consume oxygen; decreased incidence of some types of cancer; and improvement in the body's overall longevity. These benefits are supported by thousands of clinical studies.

You can no longer ignore the needs of your body. Yes, cardiovascular training is going to assist you in burning away the excess body fat, but more importantly, it is going to assist you in living an overall healthier life. One of the best gifts I have to offer you is an increase in your chances of living longer. At some point in this program, you will realize that you are participating in this program for more reasons than you thought. Somewhere along the way, you will begin to develop a personal relationship with your body. You will no longer be able to feed it with the same junk that you previously did. You will develop a deeper sense of commitment to yourself. When that happens, cardiovascular training will become one of your favorite daily activities.

It is pretty clear why I will be having you participate in a cardiovascular training program, but now it is time to discuss what we will do in order to accomplish this. Before you exercise, you will need to warm up your body and prepare it for the actual exercise. To do that, always start out with at least five minutes of walking or stretching. Once your blood is circulating faster, you can begin the actual exercise. If you decide to warm up by stretching, you will still need to warm up for at least five minutes before you start to increase the intensity of your exercise.

When you stretch, you allow your muscles to circulate more blood throughout your muscle fibers. There are many different opinions on the effectiveness of stretching before a workout, but it has not been conclusively proven that there is a benefit. I personally do not have my clients stretch before a workout, because I have never seen a clinical study that could prove that stretching reduces the chances of becoming injured. I do, however, always stretch my clients out after their workouts. I do that simply to assist in circulating some of the lactic acid that may have built up during the workout.

I have noticed some dramatic differences between the clients who stretch at the end of a workout and the clients who don't. The clients who are willing to take the extra time to properly stretch out always demonstrate fewer issues relating to soreness and fatigue. If you have already developed the habit of stretching before a workout, I encourage you to continue this habit. It is a great habit if you have the extra time; however, I have not been able to justify its need at the beginning of my workouts.

When you are warming up your body for an exercise, you are actually warming up the muscles that you will be utilizing. Some of the benefits of warming up are the prevention of a premature amount of lactic-acid buildup in your muscles; increased motor abilities; gradually building up your body's ability to consume oxygen; gradually increasing the temperature of your muscles, which can assist in avoiding injuries; allowing for a more gradual increase in your muscles' flexibility; locating possible injuries before you begin to increase the intensity of your workout; and, finally, psychologically preparing you for the exercise you will perform.

As you can see, warming up before exercise is extremely beneficial to your body's ability to adapt to the demands that you will place on it. I know that I am sounding like a personal trainer who is concerned about his clients' health, but everything that I am going to have you do has an effect on your ability to safely complete this program. Now that you have a deeper understanding of why you need to work out, we will look at the type of workout I am going to have you do.

The method of training that I have selected for this portion of the program is called continuous training. I will utilize a jogging exercise that will be stretched out over thirty minutes. The very first day you start your program, you will be required to jog for one minute and walk for twenty-nine minutes. The individuals who can already jog longer than one minute will be permitted to do so, as long as they complete the required amount of walking as well. The people who start out walking the majority of their minutes will be working toward being able to jog the entire thirty minutes by the end of the program.

Walking is a great form of exercise for those who are unable to jog, but the only people who should participate in this program are healthy individuals who are free from any medical condition that would keep them from jogging. On the last day of this program, you will be required to jog for thirty minutes nonstop. Even though I may start you out at a fast walk, I will condition you as fast as possible in order to prepare you to jog.

The reason I am so adamant about jogging is that I have always been very selective when it comes to my clients. There are many personal trainers out there, and many of them specialize in different areas of health and fitness. I have always been fascinated by quick fat-loss techniques, which is why I decided to specialize in clients who needed to get in really great shape in a very short period of time. So that I can utilize the tools that I have learned throughout the years, the clients I train have to be in good health.

If your body cannot handle jogging, this is not going to be a program for you. I hope that you will gain something from the foundation requirements, but when it comes to the exercise portion of this program, you are not going to be able to fulfill the requirements. I will not encourage anyone to complete this program who will not be able to make it through safely. If you are unable to jog, you will not be able to give yourself credit for completing the Intense Trainer Program. There are many programs out there that cater to clients with preexisting medical conditions, but this is not one of them.

I have selected jogging as the required cardiovascular exercise for this program because I have never experienced any form of exercise that can burn as many calories in a given period of time as jogging. There are different levels of intensity when it comes to jogging. Jogging is most often referred to as the next step above a fast walk, which is true; however, there are varying intensities of jogging. The definition of *jogging* in this program will be "running at a speed that is not faster than eight minutes per mile." You will not enter a sprint at any point in this program. When you enter into a sprint, you drain your body of all its energy, and you run the chance of not being able to complete your exercise for the day. If that were to happen, you would have to start over at Day 1 and work your way back up.

I have chosen a continuous exercise program because I want you to stay within your target heart rate for fat loss. If you overexert yourself, you will elevate your body past the point that it can effectively utilize stored fat as energy. If you have ever walked for an extended period of time, you know that the first time you speed up to a jog, you will usually fatigue rather quickly. The amount of exertion required to ambulate your body at a jog is almost twice the exertion that it takes to ambulate your body at a fast walk.

I first learned about the exertion difference from racehorses. A racehorse can trot for hours, but the moment you speed one up to a gallop, it tires rather quickly. There is no significant change in speed; it just requires more exertion to carry your body at a jog because there is more motion. The method by which you propel your body forward causes an increase in negative resistance against your body, which is what can often lead to lactic-acid buildup in your muscles. The more you train, the easier it will be for your body to free itself from the extra lactic-acid buildup.

I also learned from several well-known boxing trainers about the secrets they utilize to shed extra body fat from their fighters prior to fights. It is no big secret that boxers utilize the treadmill to lose weight for a fight more than any other form of exercise. The first boxing trainer I ever worked with let me in on the low-carbohydrate jogging routine. He advised me that in order for his fighters to maintain their strength when they were losing weight for a fight, he would keep their diet high in protein and low in carbohydrates. He would also withhold strength training and increase the time they spent jogging on a treadmill. It did not take me long to incorporate his techniques into my program. Much of the success of this program can be attributed to the boxing and horse-racing industries. I have utilized some of the same techniques that they have been utilizing for years, and have incorporated them into my own unique fat-loss program.

I understand that not everyone reading this program will be able to complete thirty minutes of jogging on the first day, so I have incorporated a method of training called *interval training*. Interval training combines more intense bouts of exercise with bouts of exercise that are less intense at different points within the same workout. I have decided to utilize a very successful method of getting someone who is extremely out of shape prepared to jog for thirty minutes in thirty days.

What I do is ask you to jog for the first minute and speed walk the rest of the twenty-nine minutes. On Day 2, you will jog two minutes and walk twenty-eight minutes, and so on, until you work all the way up to a thirty-minute jog. This is a very effective tool that can assist even some of the most out-of-shape clients. The minimum requirement of participants in the Intense Trainer Program is that they be able to jog for one minute and speed walk for the rest of the thirty minutes. By the end of the thirty days, you will be required to jog thirty minutes. The speed of the treadmill, or the speed of your walk, should not be that much slower than when you were jogging.

If you do not have access to a treadmill or an area to walk in, you will be required to jog in place at a fast pace. This will compensate rather well for the times that it is raining or you do not have access to a treadmill. If you thought that this program was going to be easy, you were sadly mistaken. If you are extremely overweight and somewhat discouraged about being able to complete this program, don't be. I have had several clients who weighed more than three hundred pounds when they started this program, and they were able to complete a thirty-minute jog in less than thirty days. Everything is centered on your level of commitment. If you are determined to get through the next thirty days, you will—it is that simple!

I decided to set the duration of this exercise to thirty minutes based on my past experience with clients who had difficulty losing weight. Your body does not start to fully utilize its stored fat until you have reached the twenty-minute mark. In theory, if you jog for thirty minutes, you are only burning fat for ten minutes. You will be an exception to this, because your body will already be on its way into ketosis when you start the exercise portion of this program. You will be able to start to burn fat right away. If you were on a low-fat diet, you would have to wait twenty minutes to achieve your target fat-burning zone. Please keep in mind that you will still be burning calories, even while you are waiting for your body to reach its target heart rate.

Your heart rate is the number of times your heart beats per minute. Your target heart rate is the measurement used to ensure the proper intensity of training. In order to fully maximize the number of calories you are burning during your exercise, you will want to stay within 50 to 85 percent of your maximal oxygen intake (vO2 max). The most effective way I have found to monitor this is to utilize the "talk test." The talk test gauges your ability to speak clearly during the course of your workout. If you are not able to speak clearly, that is a good indication that you are exceeding your vO2 max and need to reduce the exertion you are placing on your body. You will also want to make sure that you are pushing yourself as hard as you can without exceeding your target heart rate.

Even though you know that you will start burning fat the moment you begin exercising, you still need to condition your body to get ready to jog for thirty minutes. One of the best things that you can look forward to is knowing that in thirty days, you will already be at your most difficult level of exercise. When you go into the maintenance stage of the program, you will still be jogging only thirty minutes a day, five days a week. When you are able to jog for thirty minutes straight without stopping, however overweight you still are, I will have an extremely large amount of respect for you.

At that point, you will be able to lose all the excess body fat you want to, because you have defeated the sloth demon. It will only be a matter of time before you reach your ultimate goal. I have had some ambitious clients who wanted to jog for an hour, but I had to discourage them from doing this. If you jog long enough, you will enter an anaerobic state. When you do that, you are still burning calories, but you also stand the chance of burning valuable muscle, which is why I recommend only thirty minutes of cardiovascular exercise, no matter how in shape you are. Keep in mind that when you jog, you burn a lot of calories. When your diet is right, you will not need to burn any more than that.

As you can see, everything in this program is designed around building you up day by day. Thirty days from now, you may be shocked at the person that you have become!

Now that you know what type of exercise you will be doing, it is time to discuss strength training. Because of the importance of performing an exercise correctly, I have decided to not allow any strength-training exercises into the Intense Trainer Program. I feel that in order to properly perform any strength-training exercise, you should receive expert guidance to develop the proper form and technique. There are far too many exercises available to you for me to suggest the ones that I personally like best.

Everything in this program has to be completed exactly the way it is written. It would be far too difficult for me to safely calculate what one individual should do, because I do not know anything about his or her body. The intensity of the jogging program will be plenty sufficient to ensure maximum fat loss.

Once you have completed this program, I am going to strongly recommend that you do participate in a strength-training program, just as long as you perform it safely. I will discuss this topic in the following section.

Strength Training

The main reason that I chose not to include strength training in this program is that I do not feel you can safely include strength training into your routine unless you know how to perform the exercises properly. I recommend that you contact a personal trainer in your area who is certified by a nationally recognized certifying agency. He or she should be able to offer you the correct guidance to ensure your safety while participating in a strength-training program.

I have dedicated this section to strength training because I know that your body is going to maintain your new, higher metabolic rate much more easily when you have more lean muscle on your body. So I want to discuss some of the benefits that come along with participating in a strength-training program.

One of the first benefits is an increase in your resting metabolic rate. The muscle on your body accounts for more than 25 percent of your daily caloric expenditure. Even while you sleep, your body will be burning calories. The more muscle you add to your body, the more calories your body will burn to maintain that muscle.

Women often hesitate to start a strength-training program because they are afraid that they will bulk up. This is not a problem that you should be concerned with. A woman's body has estrogen pumping through it, not the levels of testosterone required to produce a noticeable difference in muscle size. A woman's body will just develop a more toned and firm look as a result of strength training. Lean muscle fiber is all over your body, but it is not a very thick fiber. When I am training a female client, I utilize more repetitions and smaller weights in order to ensure a leaner, more toned look.

If you are a male looking to build an abundance of muscle fiber, you will have to train with higher weights and fewer repetitions. This will prompt the tearing of muscle fibers and allow for additional growth. Whether you want to build muscle or just get toned, the bottom line is that the more muscle fiber you have, the more calories you will burn.

Another benefit of strength training is it results in a decrease in muscle-related injuries. The more developed your muscles are, the less likely you are to injure them during your daily activities. If you like to play sports, you may notice that the aches and pains that you may have felt previously will start to subside once you start a strength-training program that targets those previously aching muscles. If you like to participate in any form of physical activity that requires exertion, you will =benefit from the exercises that strengthen those parts of your body.

Professional athletes train so hard because they are trying to improve their abilities, but they are also training their bodies to be more resistant to sustaining injuries during their performance. The healthier your muscles are, the less chance you have of damaging them. If your favorite activity includes sitting on the couch and drinking beer, the only injury you are really putting yourself at risk for is pulling a muscle when you reach for the remote control. That is a sad illustration, but so many individuals would rather sit inside and watch television than go outside and have fun with their families or possibly just get some healthy oxygen pumping through their systems.

I can assure you that the more active you become, the more activities you will want to include into your day.

The third benefit of strength training I would like to point out is that when you have well-formed muscles, your body just has an overall better look. There is nothing like an appeal to vanity to underscore the need to participate in a strength-training program. The body just looks better when it is contoured with lean muscle fiber. When you are shaping your body with lean muscle, you are changing your body's entire composition.

There is no such thing as spot-reducing the amount of fat on one part of your body. This is one of the most deceptive lies that fitness-equipment manufacturers push on you. If you want a flatter stomach, you cannot get it by utilizing a certain type of abdominal machine. All you are doing when you work a particular muscle group is toning and shaping the muscle so it will be more obvious when you lose the excess body fat around it.

Making this understood is, without question, the most difficult thing that I have had to deal with when training a new client. The first thing a new client usually tells me is, "I want to tone my stomach and butt." My response to them is always the same: You will not be able to see the results until after you have lost all of the extra fat off your body. I am going to do exercises for that area of the body, not because it is going to take off the fat any sooner in that one particular area but because it will assist in the overall benefits that come along with putting more lean muscle on your body. That is why this program asks you to perform only a cardiovascular routine. Once you are able to see what it is you are training, you will gain a deeper appreciation for the benefits that come along with contouring your body with muscle.

These are just some of the reasons it is important to include strength training into your daily routine once you have successfully completed this program.

Now we will discuss some of the different methods you can utilize to add more muscle fiber to your body. One of my favorite methods of adding lean muscle is *circuit training*. Circuit training combines cardiovascular exercises with strength-building exercises. You may start out with a five-minute warm-up on the treadmill, followed by a full-body workout on circuit-training equipment. After that, you may end your workout with a thirty-minute jog on the treadmill.

Circuit-training equipment is set up to allow you to move from one piece of equipment to the next quickly enough to keep your heart rate up the entire time that you are working out. That is why I utilize it so frequently in my workout programs. If you do have the benefit of having a personal trainer, he or she should already have the next exercise ready for you to do by the time you complete the one you are performing. If you have never gotten the opportunity to experience what it feels like to work out nonstop for an hour, you should know that it is incredible. You will definitely complete your workout knowing that there is nothing more that your body can do. That is a great feeling, once you condition your body to do it. When you maintain your target heart rate the entire time you work out, you maximize the amount of fat that you are losing while you are working out. If you are training alone, circuit training will also provide you with a safer option, compared to free weights.

Another method of strength training that I utilize is known as a *dynamic workout*. In a dynamic workout, you move at an amazing pace. You do not have time to stop; you keep your body moving nonstop for approximately one hour. The main difference between circuit training and a dynamic workout is that with a dynamic workout, you always have to keep moving. This means that even while you are waiting to do the next exercise, you are jogging in place.

You also utilize light free weights when performing a dynamic workout. The main goal with a dynamic workout is to maintain an elevated heart rate for the entire workout. You also utilize more of the core exercises that are designed to strengthen your lower back, waist, and abdominal muscles. Once you have shed all of the excess body fat, you will definitely appreciate the hard work that went into sculpting your waistline. I have always liked the dynamic-workout approach, and I utilize it all the time with my clients who want a leaner, more toned appearance.

Something to keep in mind when you are putting together a dynamic workout is that you always have to know what exercise you plan to do next. If you have to think about it, you will take time away from the workout, and you run the risk of lowering your heart rate. You may want to write down the exercises that you want to do and lay out all your weights so that you can easily go from one exercise to the next. The extra time you spend preparing for this kind of workout will be well worth it once you see the results.

The third method that I will discuss is the method that I personally utilize, which includes free weights. When you include free weights in your program, you have to know how to use them correctly. Many injuries happen as a result of not performing exercises correctly. In order to work out with free weights, you need access to different amounts of weights. As you get stronger, you need to increase the demands you place on your body.

I utilize free weights because it requires more physical exertion than any other form of strength training. Once you know how to perform the exercises correctly, you will be able to safely build muscle fiber in a shorter period of time. One of the biggest drawbacks that I have found with free weights is that you need to have someone spot you when you work out.

One way I have gotten around this problem is utilizing machinery that uses free weights to add resistance. These pieces of machinery also allow you to maintain correct form, so you can always let the weight down without having a bar trap you. If you have been to a health club, you may have seen these types of apparatuses in the free-weight area. These machines can assist you in achieving the levels of strength that you are training for while maintaining your safety. If you work out at home, I always recommend working out with dumbbells. Dumbbells give you the freedom to let the weight down without being trapped by a bar.

There are many exercises you can perform just with dumbbells that will greatly benefit your body's appearance. The reason that I utilize dumbbells so frequently is that they allow me to lift heavier weights without requiring that someone spot me. If I start to get into trouble, I can always just lower the weight. If you are utilizing a bar, you can be seriously injured if you get trapped underneath it.

Once you have selected which form of strength-training exercise you want to perform, you will need to decide how long you want to work out for. It is easy to lose track of time when you are strength training. If you continue to go over your time limit, you will start to fall away from your program. I always encourage my clients to plan out the exercises that they want to perform at least one day in advance. If you are left guessing what exercises you need to perform when you get into the gym, you will never be able to maintain a consistent workout. Over time, a routine develops into a habit. Once you make a habit out of working out, it will be just as important as anything else in your life.

The important thing to keep in mind as you work out is that you always want to keep pushing yourself to the next level, which is why it is called strength training. You are trying to build as much strength as possible. Your muscle has memory and knows what you have expected from it in the past. If you start to weaken your workouts, your muscles will start to weaken as well. In order to effectively maintain a workout schedule, I recommend that you invest in a workout journal. When you keep track of your workouts and the weights that you utilized during your workouts, you will consistently make gains in your workouts. Make sure that you keep this journal in a convenient place so you can access it before and after workouts.

When you look back on the progress that you have made, you will not only see what you have accomplished but know where you are headed. The biggest advantage that this journal will give you is the ability to monitor how much time you spend working out. When you know how long it takes you to complete your workout, you will be able to structure it into your list of daily activities.

Once you start to lose the excess body fat, you will not only see the muscles that you are training, you will also feel the muscles that you are training. When you start to reduce the amount of fat covering your muscles, you will actually feel that muscle as it contracts during an exercise. The feeling that you get when you focus on a certain muscle group will serve as further validation of the good that you are doing for your body. Sure, you will feel the muscle you are exercising even when you are out of shape, but it is an entirely different story when you can feel the intensity that comes along with the swelling of that muscle.

When you supply your body with the appropriate amount of protein and nutrients, you will start to experience what is called a *muscle pump*. A muscle pump is a result of pumping more blood into a muscle than what it is normally accustomed to. A muscle pump is the equivalent to the runner's high in cardiovascular training.

The most important thing to keep in mind as your body begins to take a new shape is that you have to stay consistent with your workouts. If you do not stay consistent, you will never get a chance to fully appreciate the benefits that come along with being in great shape. Being in phenomenal shape is a result of always challenging yourself to achieve more. Over time, it will be a competition with yourself to see just how healthy you can really get. Once you start to keep track of your results, you will continue to be amazed at what you are capable of accomplishing.

When you are considering a strength-training program, you will need to consider whether you want to train in a health club or at home. Many benefits come along with joining a health club, one of which is that you have a wide variety of equipment to choose from. Another benefit is that you will have access to a fitness professional who can assist you with obtaining the correct form when you work out. One of the things I have always enjoyed about working out in a health club is the fact that if a treadmill breaks, I do not need to repair it. Once you become addicted to jogging, you will find that you need a heavy-duty treadmill.

Another added benefit of working out in a health club is that you are surrounded by people who share the same interest of getting in shape as you do. This can be a great motivating tool for the days when you are not quite in the mood to work out.

If you have children, many health clubs offer child care so that you will not be interrupted in the middle of your workout. If you like to participate in aerobics, there are usually several different classes for you to choose from at many health clubs.

I have trained in health clubs for years, and there are several reasons why I enjoy training in them. But there are also several downfalls that come along with training in a health club, one of which is equipment availability. Certain pieces of machinery may not always be available when you want them. Another inconvenience of working out in a health club is that you have to leave your house. Health clubs can be intimidating to those who do not know how a certain piece of machinery functions. They may feel clumsy or out of place if they are performing an exercise incorrectly. I have dealt with many clients who felt insecure with their bodies and did not like having people watch them exercise.

Another health-club inconvenience could be the pushy sales staff who are always attempting to sell you something. It seems that the larger the health club is, the more annoying the sales staff becomes. I have visited several clubs where the personal trainers were equally as pushy and annoying. The easiest way to deal with an annoying staff member is to wear headphones. I know from firsthand experience that I would never approach someone who was wearing headphones. By wearing headphones, you are expressing that you are serious about your workout and do not want to be bothered. This is a secret that I utilize to this day when I am visiting a gym away from my home.

If you are considering working out at home, I recommend that you consider the advantages as well as the disadvantages. One advantage of working out at home is that you do not have any excuses why you could not make it into the gym. Another advantage is that you do not have to wait for a piece of equipment to be available. You will also have the ability to work out without any unwanted attention. If you are insecure about your body, this is an important advantage. One of the things that I have always appreciated about working out at home is the convenience of not leaving my home: I can work out as hard as I want to without ever having to leave my house. I have always enjoyed working out at home, but I still occasionally train in a health club.

Something you need to consider if you do decide to strength train at home is that you will need to have the basic machinery in order to do it. I mentioned earlier that I utilize dumbbells to maximize my workouts without the assistance of a spotter, rather than utilizing free weights on a single bar. By doing this, I am able to still lift a lot of weight and do it safely. I can also load my dumbbells into my vehicle when I need to travel out of town.

Once you have selected the strength-training equipment you will need, it is time to look at cardiovascular equipment.

Because jogging will be your most common form of exercise, consider buying a treadmill. If you prefer to run outside, have a backup plan for bad weather. If you choose to work out on a treadmill, you will need to consider several factors, the first of which is what kind of treadmill to purchase. You will jog more than you will walk, so you need a heavy-duty treadmill. The treadmill should have at least a 2.5-horsepower motor, an 18-inch-wide belt, and a flexion-type system built into the floor. This will not only be more comfortable for you as you jog but will also help your treadmill last longer. You definitely do not want to purchase the cheapest treadmill on the market. I promise you that this would cause you more headaches than if you were to invest just a couple of hundred dollars more.

Another feature to look for is an accurate heart-rate monitor and calorie counter. This will make keeping track of your workout much easier. If you decide to run outside or on a track, you will need to have an alternate plan if the weather or situation does not allow you to work out: you will need to develop a good jog-in-place routine. As much as I travel, I always have to know that no matter where I am, I will be able to get in my cardiovascular workout. When I do not have access to a treadmill or the ability to jog outside, I jog in place. When you jog in place, you lift your legs higher and faster than you do when you jog on your treadmill or outside, to create the same amount of negative resistance pushing against your body. Jogging in place works great, and I usually jog in place more than any other form of cardiovascular exercise.

Once you have decided which method of training that you are going to utilize in your strength-training program, then you just need to actually do it. I can assure you that strength training will be one of the best things you can do to ensure that your metabolism does not slow down and that you will be able to maintain a healthy body for life. I hope that you will take my advice when it comes to consulting with a certified personal trainer. He or she will be able to assist you in making sure that you are performing the exercises correctly.

I have not included a strength-training program in the Intense Trainer Program because of the importance of making sure you perform the exercises properly.

I hope that you have gained a better understanding of the choices that are available to you when you decide to begin a strength-training program.

Proper Breathing

The ability to breathe properly is an absolutely essential part of completing any form of exercise. Once you understand the power that is in a breath, you will have a greater appreciation of how to properly utilize it. Did you know that you can control any emotion by the rhythm with which you choose to breathe? The techniques that I am going to share with you will not only improve your athletic performance, it will also allow you to have control over your own emotions. When you control your mood, you control your focus. Once you have focus, you will find that the exercises in this program seem effortless.

The first exercise I want to share with you is achieved by inhaling one complete breath in through your nose, and exhaling out through your mouth, utilizing your abdomen for contraction and expansion, as opposed to using your chest. Make sure that you inhale from the deepest region of your abdomen. This technique should be utilized for every exercise that you participate in. Take one deep inhale through your nose, and then complete one full exhale out through your mouth. Complete this exercise ten times before moving on to the next exercise.

Now that you have fully circulated an increased amount of oxygen through your lungs, inhale four consecutive longer breaths in through your nose, and exhale eight consecutive shorter breaths out through your mouth. Complete this exercise ten times as well. This allows your body to adjust from a very methodical pace to a more rapid pattern. As you exercise, your breathing pace will increase, and your body will adjust to an exercise better when you have properly prepared it.

Now that you have completed the first two exercises, you need to stabilize your breathing pattern. In order to do this, breathe at a pace that is conducive to the requirements you are placing on your body. If you are jogging, you need to be breathing at a pace that will supply enough oxygen to your cardiovascular system. The amount of air that your body can utilize during exercise is known as your vO2 max. The goal of any cardiovascular routine is to increase your vO2 max, so you will be able to exercise for greater periods of time without experiencing fatigue or exhaustion.

During your morning exercise, make sure that you always have the ability to speak while performing your workout. If you are not able to speak during your workout, you are not getting enough oxygen circulating throughout your cardio-vascular system. If you experience this during your workout, slow your exercising pace down until you are able to regain a normal pattern of breathing.

When you are strength training, make sure that you inhale when you are releasing the resistance and exhale during the exertion of the resistance. This will allow you to fully maximize your exertion capabilities during a workout and allow you to make substantial strength gains in a shorter period of time.

Now that you have established your breathing routine, you can use breathing as a tool to control stress and emotions. I personally developed the exercise I am going to have you complete next. If you take this exercise seriously, you will unlock a power within you that is so great that you will have to adjust to the dramatic changes over a period of time.

After experimenting with controlling stress and emotions, I looked at the possibility of using breathing to eliminate unwanted behavior. I developed this exercise when I found myself helpless when faced with negative emotions that controlled and affected my life. Have you ever had a great day, but toward the end of that great day, something or someone did something that completely ruined the happiness you had felt all day long? I am sure that everyone has experienced this at some point in their lives, but are you aware of how many times in a day your mood is affected by the circumstances around you? When you are able to stay in control and not have anyone else's actions interfere with your happiness, you are on your way to experiencing an abundant amount of peace and certainty.

You will not fully appreciate this exercise until you apply it in your everyday life. It is easy to stay calm and relaxed when you are in the privacy of your own home, but it is an entirely different story when you are out in the fast-paced world. Have you ever met someone who was absolutely calm no matter what the circumstances were? This ability is achieved when you realize that you can do only what your body will allow you to do in a certain period of time. This program will refer to this process as *pacing*.

If you have a deadline at work or you need to act quickly on a certain matter, you need to maintain a consistent pace. The only time you will experience stress is when you interrupt that pace. That is what throws you out of balance. Once that happens, you feel that you have lost control, so you speed up your actions, whether they are mental or physical. Your body does this in an effort to handle the increased demands you are placing on it.

Fear is one reaction you could have to a certain event. If you were able to maintain a consistent pace of breathing while you experienced fear, it would not be a fear at all. What happens when you become scared or you experience a large amount of anxiety? The most common reaction is to hold your breath. This very simple reaction holds the key to achieving complete control of your fears, emotions, and impulses. If you train yourself to react to fear and emotion with an exhale instead of an inhale, you will be able to successfully develop a habit that gives you complete control over your emotions.

I can tell you from firsthand experience that it is possible to retrain your mind to react with an exhale instead of an inhale, because I have done it, and so have many of my clients. I assure you that once you have successfully mastered this exercise, it will help you on the path to a life full of happiness. Your emotions will no longer be controlled by the actions of others. This is a very simple exercise, but it does require conscious effort in order to complete it.

In order for you to fully appreciate this exercise, you will need to have a greater awareness as to how your breathing affects your emotions. Right now, I want you to recall one negative experience that had a strong impact on your life. Recall that memory with as many details as possible. Notice the things that you observed, as well as the way you felt, when you were experiencing this negative emotion. Pay special attention to any sounds or smells that you may have associated with that memory. Focus on this harmful memory for at least ten minutes. Pay close attention to the way you are breathing. Do not change the way you are breathing; just observe *how* you are breathing.

Once you have completed that step, focus on a pleasant memory. Recall this memory with the same amount of detail that was in your negative memory. Make sure that you choose a memory that really brings an amazing amount of peace and happiness to you. Pay close attention to the way you are breathing. The things that you need to be looking for in your breathing pattern is how deep or how shallow your breathing is, and if your breathing is rhythmic or if it is erratic and out of balance. You need to consciously focus on how you are breathing for the entire ten minutes that you are recalling the memory.

If you performed this part of the exercise correctly, you should have noticed that when you were thinking about positive, pleasant memories, your breathing was deep and rhythmic. When you thought about the negative, unpleasant memories, you should have noticed that your breathing became shallow and erratic. What you have just experienced is absolutely crucial to the next step in this exercise. If you are not aware of how your breathing affects your emotions, you will not fully appreciate the power that comes along with training your mind to respond to unpleasant memories with a deep, consistent pattern of breathing. When you are able to face some of life's most challenging problems and still remain calm, you will create a world that is centered around the way that you want to feel, not the way life wants to make you feel.

Now that you have experienced firsthand how breathing dictates your emotions, I want you to put it to the test and see if it really does have power. Remember, a theory is something that someone states as an opinion until they are able to apply that theory and receive a noticeable outcome. So let's see if I can turn this theory into a reality for you. Right now, I want you to try to think of a very negative, harmful experience. The only catch is that you have to maintain a deep rhythm of breathing, just like the first exercise you completed. In order for you to maintain that deep rhythm, you have to focus on your breathing.

OK, let's begin! Recall a negative experience from your past, but maintain a deep rhythm of breathing. Continue to try to recall this memory as many times as you can, but continue your deep rhythm of breathing. Were you able to feel the pain from that memory? If you did, you were not focused on maintaining a deep rhythm of breathing. Most of you may have just experienced one of the most mind-altering experiences of your life. You just realized that the main thing that allows you to feel pain and discomfort is a shallow, unbalanced rhythm of breathing.

Now that you have a better understanding of how breathing affects your thoughts, it is time to utilize the tool that has completely changed not only my life but also the lives of the clients I have trained. Now, instead of recalling your negative memories with all of the details, recall the same memories in a very quick flash. As soon as you recall a negative memory, exhale. The power is within the exhale. You have the conscious ability to exhale the moment that memory is recalled.

You may have to repeat this exercise hundreds of times, but do not overlook its power. You will see and feel the benefits immediately. This is not a "hocus pocus" exercise. You will know by the end of today whether this exercise has permanently altered your reactions to the environment around you. You will be required to do this exercise throughout the entire program. By the end of this program, your life may very well never be the same. It is hard to believe that this one little exercise could produce so much happiness, but it will if you take it seriously and successfully train your mind to react with faith, instead of fear. *Faith* is the action that allows us to suffocate fear. You will understand the deeper meaning of this as you get closer to the end of the program.

The ability God gave us to control our breathing is a gift to anyone who chooses to use it. Every time you experience a thought that does not support your goals or beliefs, all you have to do is exhale. The moment a negative thought comes into your mind, just simply exhale. By the end of this program, you will have successfully retrained your mind to react with faith instead of fear. Do you remember when I discussed the importance of exhaling when you are pushing against resistance? True strength comes from the ability to exhale when faced with fear, rather than gasping for a deep breath. If this is the only thing that you take away from this entire program, it will be enough to change your life forever.

PART IV
Preparing for the Program

Program Overview

There are several elements that will factor into your ability to be successful with this program. The first is *consistency*. Without consistency, you will not properly develop a permanent habit. I have designed this program to be as simple as possible. I want you to have a clear understanding of what is required of you every day. If you are left guessing about what it is you're supposed to be doing, you will have a hard time maintaining a consistent routine throughout the entire program. The exercises I have included in this program were designed to be simple, clear, and straight to the point. The secret to developing self-discipline is the same secret that is going to allow you not only to lose a lot of body fat but also to maintain and continue to regulate the amount of body fat you have on your body for the rest of your life.

Every element of this program has three requirements you will have to meet in order to go on to the next day. If you forget even one requirement, you will be required to start over at Day 1. I am capitalizing on a psychological factor by having you do this. If you feel that you have cheated yourself even a little, you will be heading down the wrong path. It is important that you prove to yourself that you can follow directions and that you do have the ability to stick to a structured plan.

I am going to discuss each element that you will be required to complete in its entirety so that you have a clear understanding of what you will do each day.

Self-Discipline
1. Make a list of everything that you need to do today.
2. Maintain the organization of the areas that you most commonly frequent.
3. Do not allow yourself to think about anything that does not support your goals and beliefs.

You need to start your day with a list of everything you need to accomplish today. Make sure the list you make is realistic. You don't want to list anything that you know you cannot accomplish today. You have to take responsibility for everything that you list. If you are unable to accomplish one of the tasks that you have listed, you need to write down an explanation of why it was not completed today.

Place a check mark next to the scheduled task as soon as you complete it. By the end of the day, you should have successfully completed everything that is on your list. Any task that does not have a check mark should have a full explanation as to why it was not accomplished, as well as a date that it needs to be accomplished by. If for some reason one of the tasks is no longer needed, make sure that you still list the reason why it is not needed.

When you hold yourself accountable for your responsibilities, you are taking the first step toward developing self-discipline. It is easy to list something that you need to accomplish in a day, but it's an entirely different story when you have to actually complete it. This is a powerful tool to help build your self-confidence. When you look back at all of the things that you stated you were going to do, and you see that you actually did them, you will have verifiable proof that you are capable of accomplishing a task that you set out to do ahead of time. This will serve as a constant reminder of everything you are capable of accomplishing. Anyone can say that he or she can do something, but the person who actually completes it is the person who gains all of the rewards that go along with it. I cannot stress enough how important it is that you make this list and stick to it. It is vital to your success with this program.

You also need to make sure that you successfully maintain the organization of the areas around you. Your house should already be organized. If it's not, you should organize and clean it immediately. In order to maintain the organization of the areas around you, you will need to always place the items you use back in the place where they belong. Everything in your house should have a certain place where it belongs.

Organization is, without question, one of the most important factors in maintaining self-discipline. You will want to make sure that the areas that you cannot see in your house are just as organized as the areas that you can see. For example, if the common areas are organized but your closets are cluttered with the items that used to be in your common areas, you are not successfully maintaining organization.

Your mind cannot properly function when there is chaos all around you. You are creating a sensory overload of your mind. How can you expect to feel as if you are in control of your personal environment when everything around you is in a disorganized state? If your life is not organized, it will be by the end of this program. When you are competing against the game of life, you are competing against a stacked deck, and you have to put as many odds back in your corner as you possibly can.

The first step is to ensure that everything around you has a place where it belongs. I understand that if you have kids, it is going to be difficult to maintain a sense of organization in your house, but it is possible. There is no time like the present to pass these gifts on to your children. If your children grow up knowing that they have to maintain the organization of the areas around them, they will be ten steps ahead of most children.

If you are not already organized, I want you to make sure that you are organized before you start this program. This is a requirement that must be completed every day in order for you to qualify as having completed the program. You will thank me once you get to see the results of staying organized. Your mind will be able to think much more clearly. This one exercise has the ability to dramatically enhance your lifestyle. I hope that you will treat it seriously and act on it today. Make sure that you do not even think about trying to start this program without a sense of organization—it is that important.

You need to ensure that your thoughts are supporting your goals and beliefs. You already know that any thought that does not support your goal will create doubt over time. You must maintain absolute focus at all times. As soon as a thought comes into your head that does not support your goals or beliefs, you must redirect that thought to the things that do support your goals and beliefs. This technique will prevent doubt from even starting. Remember, one thought directs another thought until it produces a noticeable outcome. If you are thinking about things that do not support your goals, you may not fail immediately, but in time your negative thoughts will gain momentum, and before you know it, you will have failed.

The ability to discipline your thoughts is the foundation of self-discipline. Disciplining your thoughts does require effort, so you must always be ready to defend your newly established beliefs. You will always be in control of your thoughts and actions once you're able to interrupt the negative thought process before it even has a chance to produce a noticeable outcome.

In order for you to redirect your thoughts, you first have to be aware of your thoughts. This is often a very uncomfortable experience. It can almost be a burden to you if you have not ever consciously paid attention to your thoughts and internal dialogue. You have self-talk throughout the entire day. You just may not be aware of what you're telling yourself.

If all that you are thinking about is what makes you upset, or what you would rather be doing instead of accomplishing a certain task, your thoughts and actions will be in a state of constant conflict. You will be telling yourself one thing while you expect to achieve something else. For example, you want to lose body fat, so you decide to start this program. But all you're able to think about is everything you're missing out on by restricting certain foods from your diet. Do you honestly think that you will be able to stay seriously committed to a program that is depriving you of the foods that you would rather be eating? It has been my experience that you won't.

Your thoughts have to be congruent with your goals and beliefs. If they are not, you will eventually fail this program. There is no way around that. At the end of this program, you will gain a better understanding of the importance of this exercise.

The first time you start to think about something that goes against your goal of completing this program, you will have to redirect that thought immediately. It's that simple. It will be difficult at first, but you will find that after a few days, this exercise will start to bring you a lot of happiness. This one exercise has the ability to dramatically enhance your quality of life, so please take it seriously.

Now that we have discussed the importance of the three elements you will be utilizing to establish and build self-discipline, let's discuss your diet. Your daily diet requirements are set in stone as far as this program is concerned. There will be no room for flexibility whatsoever. You will be required to complete each exercise every single day of this program. I have really focused on developing a program that is as strict as it can possibly be without jeopardizing your health.

Again, I urge you to consult with your doctor before participating in any part of this program. If you are not healthy, you could endanger your health and well-being. I care about you, and I want to make sure that you make it through this program safely.

Diet
1. Make a list of all the foods you're going to eat today.
2. List all of the calories and carbohydrates in the meals you consume.
3. Do not exceed your daily caloric and carbohydrate allowance.

In order to ensure your success with this program, you will need to pay close attention to the foods you consume. You need to make a list of all the foods you intend to eat. If you do not have a guideline, you run the risk of not having the appropriate foods ready when it's time for you to eat. When you write out a list ahead of time, it will also allow you to establish your food-intake parameters for the day. By having a list to refer to, you will actually create more spare time to concentrate on other areas of your life.

If someone asks you whether you would like something to eat, you will be able to say no, because you will know it's not on your list. If they should happen to have something that is on your list, feel free to enjoy that meal or snack.

A list is crucial in establishing your daily dietary parameters. If you are left guessing what you can or cannot eat, you will find yourself in a situation that may compromise your dietary parameters. One of the most common reasons for dietary failure is not having a clear set of parameters. You should be able to know immediately if you can or cannot eat a certain type of food.

During the first week of this program, this will be a somewhat difficult task. Once you establish a clear guideline as to what you can eat, it will allow you to focus on the other elements of this program. If someone approaches you, especially a family member, you have to be ready with a response as to why you cannot eat a certain type of food. If you have the support of your family through this program, it will greatly increase your odds of completing it. If someone offers you cake or any other food that may tempt you, you have to respond quickly to their offer. A quick no will suffice just fine. If they seem eager with their advance, you will need to let them know that you are serious about completing this program, and that you do not want the food they are offering you.

In my past, this has never failed: someone would approach me with one of my favorite foods at a time when I was feeling a lot of unwanted tension about dieting. If I did not respond with a quick no, it seemed as if that person could sense that I wanted the food he or she was offering me, and he or she would try that much harder to get me to eat a food that I knew I could not have on my diet. When someone senses that you are struggling with your self-esteem, they may try to sabotage you. It is a primal function that allows them to keep you on their level. Who wants someone to become stronger than him or her? Very few people.

You will have to stay committed to your list so that you will not be tempted to cheat; it's that simple. Don't make it any more complex than it really is. If a food is not on your list, you cannot eat it.

As soon as you complete a meal, you need to write down the exact number of calories and carbohydrates in that meal. If you do not write down the number of calories or carbohydrates, you may find at the end of the day that you went over your daily allowance. If that were to happen, you would be required to start over at the beginning of the program. Even though it may seem like a chore at first, you will definitely learn the benefits of calculating your daily intake totals. It is very easy to forget about five or six grams of carbohydrates. Please remember that if you consume more than twenty grams of carbohydrates, you run the risk of ending your state of ketosis. The twenty-carbohydrate limit exists for a reason.

The caloric and carbohydrate allowance we have established is not flexible. It has to be maintained without any breach in parameters in order to ensure your success with this program.

There is nothing worse than adding up your calorie and carbohydrate totals at the end of your day only to find that you went over your daily limit. This can be very frustrating. When you write down the exact number of calories and carbohydrates that are in the meals you consume immediately after you consume it, you will know before the end of the day whether you are getting close to your daily limits. You should know at lunchtime whether you are on track with your limits.

This will seem like a tedious requirement at first, but when you complete this program, you will have developed a habit of always keeping a mental total in your head that will allow you to maintain your fat loss once you have completed this program. I have had several days in my past where I thought I did so well, only to find that I forgot to add in a snack that I had at the beginning of the day. You will want to eat every gram of energy you're allowed. It almost becomes a mathematical game that you play with yourself. I love to calculate my total at night, because when I'm able to lay my head on my pillow knowing that I completed what I said I was going to complete, an amazing feeling comes along with that. I encourage you to take this exercise very seriously. It will be difficult at first, but in time it will give you pleasure when you're able to add up your total and know that you did a good job. There's nothing like positive motivation that comes from yourself.

Not exceeding your daily dietary allowance is not only important for your fat-loss success but also for your ability to maintain self-discipline. If you go over your daily allowance even by ten calories, you run the risk of losing the level of self-discipline you have established up to this point. Maintaining your dietary-allowance parameters may be one of the most crucial elements that will ensure your successful completion of this program. The most common reason people are unable to stay under their daily allowance is that they do not write down their intake totals when they complete a meal. If you rely on your memory to calculate your intake totals, you will more than likely end up going over your daily allowance at some point in this program. Your ability to maintain momentum is crucial to the success of this program. Stay focused and do not exceed your dietary allowance.

Exercise
1. Jog the required minutes, then walk the required minutes at a fast pace.
2. Start your exercise within the first hour that you are awake.
3. Drink 16 ounces of water before and after your workout.

The first day of the program, you will be required to jog at least one minute. If you are capable of jogging for longer than that, you need to put forth the extra effort and jog for as long as you can. You want to make sure that you do not over-exert yourself, because you could run the risk of not being able to complete the required minutes of walking. Every day, you should be challenging yourself to jog longer. If you are out of shape, you will appreciate the gradual increase in jogging, but if you are already capable of jogging for extended periods of time, you will need to keep challenging yourself.

I decided to start you out with a one-minute minimum because I want to give someone who is out of shape a chance to successfully complete this program. If I were to require everyone to jog for thirty minutes, I would only have a handful of people who could complete this program. I have designed the exercise portion of this program with the same concept that I have used throughout the entire program: start out small, and work your way up.

When you are required to jog an additional minute every day, you will build up the stamina to handle thirty minutes by the end of the program. The cardiovascular system is absolutely amazing in how quickly it responds to cardiovascular exercises. A person who is having difficulty breathing on the first workout may find that in ten days, he or she is able to breathe with ease during the entire workout.

I like to elevate your heart rate as quickly as possible so I can maximize the amount of time you're actually burning fat. If you are capable of jogging longer than the minimum requirement, you had better be putting forth the additional effort to make sure that it happens. If you choose to be lazy when you know that you are capable of more, you're only cheating yourself. I hope that you will exercise balance when completing your workouts, and that you will not overexert yourself to the point at which you cannot complete the walking portion of your workout. When you are able to balance pushing yourself hard with still completing your workout, you will know that you are well on your way to becoming physically fit. The exercise portion of this program is required in order for your body to burn stored fat.

I have already stressed the importance of exercising within the first hour that you are awake; it is a requirement needed to successfully complete this program. You must be able to start your day one step ahead of the game. If you are planning to exercise at the end of your day, you will miss a workout. I have been training clients for years, and I have never seen someone consistently work out every night when they got off work. There will be times when something will come up, and you will have to put off a workout. You have to eliminate this problem from ever being a factor in this program.

You will be required to exercise every day for the next thirty days. If you miss even one workout, you will have to start over from the beginning. We have already discussed how the completion percentage is reduced after the first attempt. It takes discipline to just jump out of bed and work out, but that's one of the elements we're training. There are just too many factors that can interfere with your ability to get in a workout. If you do not work out within the first hour that you are awake, the chances of you completing this program are very slim.

Remember, you need to add as many tools to your arsenal as possible. By working out first thing in the morning, you're giving yourself the opportunity to succeed within the first hour that you are awake. I hope that you will take this exercise requirement seriously. I had to add it because it is absolutely crucial to your success.

I require sixteen ounces of water before you exercise, and sixteen ounces after you exercise, because you are not capable of properly monitoring the amount of fluid your body needs during your workout. If you were to rely on thirst to let you know when you needed to consume more fluids, your body would always be 50 to 75 percent dehydrated. Your body does not have a way of telling you how much water you need to consume during exercise, because you're burning calories at a significantly increased rate. When this happens, the only method you have of preparing your body for the increased demand is to hydrate your body before and after your workout.

The water you consume before and after your workout is in addition to the water you need to consume throughout the day. After you have completed your workout, you should consume at least thirty-two ounces more throughout your day. I promise you that when you see the results that come along with consuming this much water, you will thank me. Your body needs every advantage it can get when you're breaking down a significant amount of body fat. Your water intake should continue at this level even after you have completed this program. As with the other elements of this program, you will be required to complete these steps every day of the program. If you miss even one exercise, you will be required to start over at the beginning of the program.

Now that you know what is expected of you every day, it's time to look at the things you will need to have in place before starting this program. The first is a place where you can exercise. You need to know exactly where you are going to jog every day. If you are going to be exercising on a treadmill, you will need to make arrangements to either own one or have guaranteed access to one for the entire thirty days. If you plan on exercising outside, you need to have a backup plan in case the weather does not cooperate with you. Jogging in place should always be the default mode if you are unable to get to a treadmill or outside. I have spent many mornings in a hotel jogging in place because I did not have access to a treadmill. One thing to keep in mind is that if you do jog in place, you will have to move at a faster pace than if you were actually traveling a distance.

Now that you have your method of exercise established, you need to make sure that you stock up on all of the foods you will be consuming for the next week. There is nothing worse than trying to adjust to a new method of eating and finding yourself stuck at lunchtime without food that you can eat. You'll only be setting yourself up for disaster if you are relying on eating out or going to the grocery store every day. Make sure that you make the first week of this program as easy as possible.

In addition to all the necessary foods, you need to have the proper vitamin supplementation. You can find the appropriate vitamin at just about any reputable pharmacy or grocery store. Usually the vitamins that cater toward low-carbohydrate diets are the best for this program. Read the directions carefully, and make sure the vitamin will provide you with the appropriate nutrients.

While you're at the pharmacy picking up your vitamins, you can ask your pharmacist for ketone-testing strips. Make sure you get the testing strips that offer several different levels of ketone fluctuation. You will appreciate this when you are indicating a large amount of ketones in your system. It will serve as further validation that your body is burning fat at a very rapid pace.

OK, now you have all of the necessary tools to ensure your success. The last thing that you need to do is a get a good night's sleep. You want to make sure that you are well rested, because the next thirty days will absolutely shape the rest of your life. Make sure that your body is just as prepared as your mind. Once you awake from your sound sleep, make sure that you start your workout as quickly as possible. It will take only a few days to get your body used to this type of change. Once your body has adjusted to it, you will actually start to look forward to your morning workouts. Sleep well, and we will start the first day of the program when you're ready. Be strong, and you're going to do just fine.

Measuring Body Composition

I will never agree with or support any fat-loss program that utilizes your body weight as an accurate method of determining your body's composition. If you were to go by the older, traditional methods of determining body composition, I would be considered morbidly obese, and I have only 6 percent body fat.

You will analyze the results you receive from this program by a set of measurements: of your upper right arm, waistline, hips, and upper right thigh. I have had many clients lose a substantial number of inches from their waistlines and still only weigh a few pounds less than when started.

Lean muscle weighs almost twice as much as fat. You cannot overlook this amazing fact. The more lean muscle you have on your body, the more calories your body will burn. I have already discussed the effect lean muscle has on the metabolism, but it's also important to point out that lean muscle does weigh substantially more than fat. If you decide that you absolutely have to weigh yourself before you start Day 1 of this program, that's fine, but under no circumstances will you be permitted to weigh yourself until the last day of the program. I have had many clients fail this program because of the jaded perception that a scale gave them. I'm going out of my way to make sure that you fully understand that a scale will have a very negative impact on your success in this program. I would prefer that you throw away any scale that you may have, and never use a scale to determine your body composition again.

I have observed several well-known weight-loss programs utilizing weight as the primary tool for determining the success of their program. What they do not tell you is that the majority of people who complete their program end up gaining more weight back once they eventually fail to abide by the parameters of the diet. These misguided individuals thought that they were losing a lot of fat, only to realize that they had ended up losing precious muscle fiber that would have allowed them to return to a more flexible meal plan once they were at their desired goal. If you decide to lose just weight, any of these weight-loss programs will suffice, but if you want a healthy, lean, and toned body, you will need to follow the parameters of this program.

On Day 1 of this program, I am going to have you measure various parts of your body. The first part of the body that I will ask you to measure is your upper right arm. I chose the right arm because I want you to measure only one side of your body. No one has a perfectly symmetrical body. By taking only one measurement from your right side, you can properly obtain an accurate determination of your fat loss.

Make sure to use a soft and flexible cloth measuring tape. Once you have the proper measuring tape, measure the area of the upper arm that is located between the shoulder and the elbow. Make sure that the tape is laid across the arm, not pulled tight. If you rely on getting the tape tight, you will never be able to record an accurate measurement. The measuring tape should be no more than slightly snug.

Once you have this measurement, record it in the appropriate section on Day 1 of this program. You will not take another measurement until Day 30. I know it will be tempting at times, but you need to make sure that the results you see in thirty days will excite you enough to stay committed to relying on measurements instead of weight for the rest of your life.

The next part of the body that I'm going to have you measure is your waistline. This measurement is taken by placing the measuring tape around your waist and across your navel. Make sure that the measuring tape does not slip lower or higher on your back than it is across your navel. It will throw your measurement off by inches if you do not make sure that the tape is perfectly flat and in a straight line all the way around your waist. Once the tape is just barely snug, you will want to record that measurement in the appropriate section of Day 1.

After you have recorded your waistline measurement, record your hip measurement. Place the measuring tape around the center region of your buttocks and pull the tape around to the center of your groin area. Once you have obtained an accurate measurement, you need to record it in the appropriate section of Day 1.

The last measurement that you need to record is your upper-right-thigh measurement. Place the measuring tape around the upper region of your thigh, located between your groin and knee. After you have determined the accurate measurement, you need to record it in the appropriate section of Day 1.

Now that you have recorded all of the required measurements, it is time to put that measuring tape away for thirty days. On Day 30 of this program, you will record these measurements again. I hope that you will appreciate the results you receive from being patient and waiting until the last day of this program to examine your results. It will give you even more of a reason to celebrate.

If you decide that you have to weigh in on the first day, make sure that you do not weigh yourself again until the last day of this program. Once you have reached your dream physique, all you have to do is maintain those measurements for life. Instead of being upset by a fluctuating scale, you will be able to rely on measurements that allow you to maintain the perfect body, not the perfect weight.

Final Checklist

Now that you are getting closer to the point when you will be ready to start Day 1 of this program, you need to make sure that you are able to check off everything on this list. If you decide to start Day 1 when you know that you do not have everything on this list, you are setting yourself up for failure before you even start. I hope you will take this list seriously. Do not under any circumstance start this program until everything on this list is present and accounted for. I congratulate you for getting this far. Every requirement I have put in place is to help you successfully complete this program. I hope that you can see that, and I look forward to starting Day 1 with you when you are ready!

You need:

1.   The belief that you will be able to complete this program

2.   The appropriate foods for your diet

3.   The proper ketone testing strips

4.   Access to a treadmill or other jogging arrangements

5.   A signed personal agreement.

Personal Agreement

Whenever you commit to something in writing, you will always have a better chance of accomplishing it. I'm sure by now you have already gained a better understanding of that, so we will proceed on to the personal-agreement section of this program. By signing a personal agreement to yourself, you are binding yourself by personal law to abide by the commitment you make to yourself. The only person who will suffer the consequences of breaking this agreement is you.

I assure you that if you do break this agreement, you will have a difficult time recovering from it. The chances of you successfully completing this program the second time around are very slim. You have to make sure that you are 100 percent committed to taking on the responsibility of completing every exercise in this program. If you fail to even complete one exercise, you will have breached the agreement, and you will fall that much further away from ever being able to successfully lose all of your excess body fat.

If you are not ready to take these exercises seriously, you are not ready to commit to the following agreement, and I strongly advise you to not sign this agreement. I already know the devastating consequences someone goes through when he or she is not able to complete this agreement. But if you feel that you are willing to commit to this program with 100 percent of your focus and attention, you will be ready to sign this agreement and start Day 1.

Please read the following agreement carefully, and sign it when you are ready.

I, _____, hereby agree to all of the terms in this program.

      (print your name)

I will successfully complete every exercise in its entirety, and will execute them to the best of my ability. Under no circumstances other than medically related issues will I breach this agreement. I am signing this agreement because I know that I am ready to complete this entire program over the next thirty days. I am making a personal promise to myself that for once in my life, I will not succumb to the impulses that caused me to store excess body fat. I understand that if I do not complete every exercise in its entirety, I will be required to start over at Day 1, and I will have broken the promise I made to myself today.

_____

(signature)(today's date)

PART V
Daily Exercises

DAY 1

Self-Discipline
1. Make a list of everything that you need to do today.
2. Maintain the organization of the areas that you most commonly frequent.
3. Do not allow yourself to think about anything that does not support your goals and beliefs.

Diet
1. Make a list of all the foods you're going to eat today.
2. List all of the calories and carbohydrates in the meals you consume.
3. Do not exceed your daily caloric and carbohydrate allowance.

Exercise
1. Jog at least 1 minute, then walk 29 minutes at a fast pace.
2. Start your exercise within the first hour that you are awake.
3. Drink 16 ounces of water before and after your workout.

Daily Expectations

Today you can expect to have some minor cravings, probably closer to the time you go to sleep. Your body still has plenty of carbohydrates in its system, so you will not be experiencing any unusual cravings at this point. The largest obstacle you will have to face today is a change in your normal eating routine. Whenever you change a routine, you will have to make adjustments. Instead of grabbing a piece of cake, you will be grabbing a piece of meat.

Today is actually one of the easiest days in the program, because you are more than likely excited to lose the fat and will not be as tempted to consume carbohydrates as in the days to come. You can expect your energy level to be the same as it has been up to this point. You may even have more energy than normal from the excitement of losing all of your excess body fat.

Your ketone test strip will probably not indicate any ketones at this point, unless you restricted carbohydrates before you started this program.

Please keep in mind that you have twenty-nine days left, so you need to pace your energy level. Congratulations on taking the first step toward permanently enhancing your health and physique. I will be including a new set of daily expectations with every passing day. They will serve as a reminder of the things you can expect to deal with as you start that specific day. Each day will have its own unique challenges. If you're prepared for them, you will be able to overcome them a lot easier. I want you to stay focused and maintain that determination that has gotten you this far. Make sure that you monitor your breathing and complete every exercise required.

Day 1

Date _____ / _____ / _____

Daily caloric-intake limit: _____ Daily carbohydrate limit: 20

Provide your body-composition measurements

Right upper arm: _____ Waistline: _____ Hips: _____ Right upper thigh: _____

List everything that you need to accomplish today

_____

_____

_____

_____

_____

List the foods that you intend to consume today

_____

_____

_____

_____

_____

List the caloric and carbohydrate totals from the foods you consumed

Food source: _____ Caloric total: _____ Carbohydrate total: ___

Food source: _____ Caloric total: _____ Carbohydrate total: ___

Food source: _____ Caloric total: _____ Carbohydrate total: ___

Food source: _____ Caloric total: _____ Carbohydrate total: ___

Food source: _____ Caloric total: _____ Carbohydrate total: ___

Food source: _____ Caloric total: _____ Carbohydrate total: ___

Food source: _____ Caloric total: _____ Carbohydrate total: ___

Food source: _____ Caloric total: _____ Carbohydrate total: ___

Food source: _____ Caloric total: _____ Carbohydrate total: ___

Food source: _____ Caloric total: _____ Carbohydrate total: ___

Daily caloric total: _____ Daily carbohydrate total: _____

List the amount of minutes you were able to jog and walk

Jog: _____ Walk: _____

Place a check mark next to your current ketone level

None: _____ Trace: _____ Moderate: _____ Large: _____ High: _____

DAY 2

Self-Discipline
1. Make a list of everything that you need to do today.
2. Maintain the organization of the areas that you most commonly frequent.
3. Do not allow yourself to think about anything that does not support your goals and beliefs.

Diet
1. Make a list of all the foods that you will eat today.
2. List all of the calories and carbohydrates in the meals you consume.
3. Do not exceed your daily caloric and carbohydrate allowance.

Exercise
1. Jog at least 2 minutes, then walk 28 minutes at a fast pace.
2. Start your exercise within the first hour that you are awake.
3. Drink 16 ounces of water before and after your workout.

Daily Expectations

Today you can expect to have food cravings toward the end of the day. You may notice that you find yourself eating more than usual. Your body is starting to sense that carbohydrates are being restricted. As a result, you may find yourself wanting to consume more food than usual. When you begin to eat a meal, you need to have available only the portion of food that you intend to eat. If you still feel hungry when you complete your meal, wait twenty minutes. You will find that if you wait just twenty minutes, the cravings will diminish.

Today is going to be somewhat difficult, because your body is preparing to convert over to utilizing ketone bodies for energy. When you exercise, you will still have plenty of energy to complete your workout. If you can jog for a longer period of time, do so. Make sure that you stay consistent with these exercises. Every day, you are required to complete every exercise. Make sure that you do not have to start over.

Your ketone test strip may possibly show a trace of ketone bodies. Some of my clients have shown a moderate to large amount of ketones on the second day of training. If you do indicate more than a trace amount, that just means you're that much closer to losing all of your excess body fat. Make sure that you keep your momentum going. And last but not least, make sure that you monitor your breathing and complete every exercise required. You have to stay strong in order to complete just twenty-eight more days. In only a couple of days, things are going to get much easier. Just keep going!

Day 2

Date: _____ / _____ / _____

Daily caloric-intake limit: _____ Daily carbohydrate limit: 20

List everything that you need to accomplish today

_____
_____
_____
_____
_____

List the foods that you intend to consume today

_____
_____
_____
_____
_____

List the caloric and carbohydrate totals from the foods you consumed

Food source: _____ Caloric total: _____ Carbohydrate total: ___
Food source: _____ Caloric total: _____ Carbohydrate total: ___
Food source: _____ Caloric total: _____ Carbohydrate total: ___
Food source: _____ Caloric total: _____ Carbohydrate total: ___
Food source: _____ Caloric total: _____ Carbohydrate total: ___
Food source: _____ Caloric total: _____ Carbohydrate total: ___
Food source: _____ Caloric total: _____ Carbohydrate total: ___
Food source: _____ Caloric total: _____ Carbohydrate total: ___
Food source: _____ Caloric total: _____ Carbohydrate total: ___
Food source: _____ Caloric total: _____ Carbohydrate total: ___

Daily caloric total: _____ Daily carbohydrate total: _____

List the amount of time you were able to jog and walk

Jog: _____ Walk: _____

Place a check mark next to your current ketone level

None: _____ Trace: _____ Moderate: _____ Large: _____ High: _____

DAY 3

Self-Discipline
1. Make a list of everything that you need to do today.
2. Maintain the organization of the areas that you most commonly frequent.
3. Do not allow yourself to think about anything that does not support your goals and beliefs.

Diet
1. Make a list of all the foods that you will eat today.
2. List all of the calories and carbohydrates in the meals you consume.
3. Do not exceed your daily caloric and carbohydrate allowance.

Exercise
1. Jog at least 3 minutes, then walk 27 minutes at a fast pace.
2. Start your exercise within the first hour that you are awake.
3. Drink 16 ounces of water before and after your workout.

Daily Expectations

Today may be one of the most difficult days you will face in the entire program. You may notice that your energy is somewhat low. You will need to force yourself through this stage. Your body is well on its way into ketosis, and you will feel the effects of converting over to ketone bodies for energy.

Today you will need to pay close attention to your discipline exercises. Make sure that your thoughts support you in completing this program. Make sure that you begin your exercise within the first hour that you are awake. You will need the extra energy that you have stored from your night's sleep in order to ensure that you complete your workout.

This morning, your ketone test strip may indicate a moderate to large amount of ketones. The levels of ketones indicated in your test strip are a direct reflection of the amount of carbohydrates you had in your system prior to beginning the program. If you pigged out on carbohydrates before you started this program, it will take longer for your body to show the presence of ketones.

The advantage of being challenged for energy is that you will realize that energy is nothing more than a state of mind. If you feel run-down today, you will need to force yourself to act with more energy. This exercise will allow you to see that your body and mind can function just as well, if not better, on ketones. Whatever you do today, make sure that you stay strong. Make sure that you monitor your breathing and complete every exercise required. You are almost past the most difficult stage of this program. Keep going!

Day 3

Date: _____ / _____ / _____

Daily caloric-intake limit: _____ Daily carbohydrate limit: 20

List everything that you need to accomplish today

_____

_____

_____

_____

_____

List the foods that you intend to consume today

_____

_____

_____

_____

_____

List the caloric and carbohydrate totals from the foods you consumed

Food source: _____ Caloric total: _____ Carbohydrate total: ___

Food source: _____ Caloric total: _____ Carbohydrate total: ___

Food source: _____ Caloric total: _____ Carbohydrate total: ___

Food source: _____ Caloric total: _____ Carbohydrate total: ___

Food source: _____ Caloric total: _____ Carbohydrate total: ___

Food source: _____ Caloric total: _____ Carbohydrate total: ___

Food source: _____ Caloric total: _____ Carbohydrate total: ___

Food source: _____ Caloric total: _____ Carbohydrate total: ___

Food source: _____ Caloric total: _____ Carbohydrate total: ___

Food source: _____ Caloric total: _____ Carbohydrate total: ___

Daily caloric total: _____ Daily carbohydrate total: _____

List the amount of time you were able to jog and walk

Jog: _____ Walk: _____

Place a check mark next to your current ketone level

None: _____ Trace: _____ Moderate: _____ Large: _____ High: _____

DAY 4

Self-Discipline
1. Make a list of everything that you need to do today.
2. Maintain the organization of the areas that you most commonly frequent.
3. Do not allow yourself to think about anything that does not support your goals and beliefs.

Diet
1. Make a list of all the foods that you will eat today.
2. List all of the calories and carbohydrates in the meals you consume.
3. Do not exceed your daily caloric and carbohydrate allowance.

Exercise
1. Jog at least 4 minutes, then walk 26 minutes at a fast pace.
2. Start your exercise within the first hour that you are awake.
Drink 16 ounces of water before and after your workout.

Daily Expectations

Today is going to be a relatively challenging day as well. The good news is that your body should already be converted completely over to utilizing ketone bodies for energy. When you eat your meals, you will want to make sure that you do not consume more than what is on the plate in front of you. Your body is still craving carbohydrates. The moment you begin to consume your meal, your body may react with an amazing amount of hunger. This is a fairly common experience on the fourth day of this program.

If you wait just twenty minutes, this intense craving will subside. You need to exercise self-discipline in order to keep from eating more than what is in front of you. Once you make it through that twenty-minute time span, you will experience firsthand how to defeat a craving. Once your body realizes that you have assumed total control over the foods you are going to eat, these intense cravings will disappear altogether.

Today your ketone test strip should indicate that you have a moderate to large amount of ketones. If your test strip does not indicate a moderate amount of ketones in your system, you are consuming too many carbohydrates. You need to make sure that you are monitoring the ingredients in your meals a lot more closely. If you are not in ketosis by tomorrow, we may have a problem.

Stay strong and focus on your ability to overcome the cravings you have demolished today. When you get a craving to do something and override that feeling with an action that supports your belief, you will begin to gain a lot of strength from that. Over the next twenty-six days, you will start to fully appreciate the strength and power that comes from taking control of your body. Make sure that you monitor your breathing and complete every exercise required. You have almost made it through the toughest portion of the program, so stay focused and keep going!

Day 4

Date: _____ / _____ / _____

Daily caloric-intake limit: _____ Daily carbohydrate limit: 20

List everything that you need to accomplish today

_____

_____

_____

_____

_____

List the foods that you intend to consume today

_____

_____

_____

_____

_____

List the caloric and carbohydrate totals from the foods you consumed

Food source: _____ Caloric total: _____ Carbohydrate total: ___

Food source: _____ Caloric total: _____ Carbohydrate total: ___

Food source: _____ Caloric total: _____ Carbohydrate total: ___

Food source: _____ Caloric total: _____ Carbohydrate total: ___

Food source: _____ Caloric total: _____ Carbohydrate total: ___

Food source: _____ Caloric total: _____ Carbohydrate total: ___

Food source: _____ Caloric total: _____ Carbohydrate total: ___

Food source: _____ Caloric total: _____ Carbohydrate total: ___

Food source: _____ Caloric total: _____ Carbohydrate total: ___

Food source: _____ Caloric total: _____ Carbohydrate total: ___

Daily caloric total: _____ Daily carbohydrate total: _____

List the amount of time you were able to jog and walk

Jog: _____ Walk: _____

Place a check mark next to your current ketone level

None: _____ Trace: _____ Moderate: _____ Large: _____ High: _____

DAY 5

Self-Discipline
1. Make a list of everything that you need to do today.
2. Maintain the organization of the areas that you most commonly frequent.
3. Do not allow yourself to think about anything that does not support your goals and beliefs.
Diet
1. Make a list of all the foods that you will eat today.
2. List all of the calories and carbohydrates in the meals you consume.
3. Do not exceed your daily caloric and carbohydrate allowance.
Exercise
1. Jog at least 5 minutes, then walk 25 minutes at a fast pace.
2. Start your exercise within the first hour that you are awake.
3. Drink 16 ounces of water before and after your workout.

Daily Expectations

Today you will notice that your hunger cravings are subsiding. Your body is now utilizing stored fat for energy, and it has already made the transition into ketosis. You will find that controlling your caloric and carbohydrate limits will begin to get easier.

The one element that you still need to watch for is when you begin to eat a meal; your body may still have a reaction and want you to eat more. This will be gone soon, but you need to be prepared to defeat this craving. For many years, you probably ate the moment that you felt hungry. Now you are relying on yourself to make the decision when you are going to eat. This transition takes some getting used to, but the results last a lifetime. Once you prove to yourself that you are capable of having control over the cravings, your body will cease to have them. This is definitely a mental element that is being corrected as we speak. You have to keep the momentum going and make sure that you are waiting twenty minutes after your meals to properly determine your hunger.

Your ketone test strip should be indicating a moderate to large amount of ketones.

You defeated the most challenging aspect of this program the moment you took back control of your hunger. Now you just need to stay focused and make sure that you are completing your self-discipline exercises. Make sure that you monitor your breathing and complete every exercise required. You're doing great—keep going!

Day 5

Date: _____ / _____ / _____

Daily caloric-intake limit: _____ Daily carbohydrate limit: 20

List everything that you need to accomplish today

_____
_____
_____
_____
_____

List the foods that you intend to consume today

_____
_____
_____
_____
_____

List the caloric and carbohydrate totals from the foods you consumed

Food source: _____ Caloric total: _____ Carbohydrate total: ___
Food source: _____ Caloric total: _____ Carbohydrate total: ___
Food source: _____ Caloric total: _____ Carbohydrate total: ___
Food source: _____ Caloric total: _____ Carbohydrate total: ___
Food source: _____ Caloric total: _____ Carbohydrate total: ___
Food source: _____ Caloric total: _____ Carbohydrate total: ___
Food source: _____ Caloric total: _____ Carbohydrate total: ___
Food source: _____ Caloric total: _____ Carbohydrate total: ___
Food source: _____ Caloric total: _____ Carbohydrate total: ___
Food source: _____ Caloric total: _____ Carbohydrate total: ___

Daily caloric total: _____ Daily carbohydrate total: _____

List the amount of time you were able to jog and walk

Jog: _____Walk: _____

Place a check mark next to your current ketone level

None: _____ Trace: _____ Moderate: _____ Large: _____ High: _____

DAY 6

Self-Discipline

1. Make a list of everything that you need to do today.

2. Maintain the organization of the areas that you most commonly frequent.

3. Do not allow yourself to think about anything that does not support your goals and beliefs.

Diet

1. Make a list of all the foods that you will eat today.

2. List all of the calories and carbohydrates in the meals you consume.

3. Do not exceed your daily caloric and carbohydrate allowance.

Exercise

1. Jog at least 6 minutes, then walk 24 minutes at a fast pace.

2. Start your exercise within the first hour that you are awake.

3. Drink 16 ounces of water before and after your workout.

Daily Expectations

Today will be a great day! You should notice that almost all of your cravings are gone and that your workouts are becoming easier. By now, you may notice that you do have control over your cravings, and you do not really need to eat as much as you may have thought. This is a great side effect of being in ketosis. You are no longer dealing with surges of insulin, and your mind is able to override your feelings of hunger.

Now that the dust is starting to settle, you need to remain focused. From this point on, the program only becomes easier. But you will want to keep in mind that you are only a thought away from losing it. The first time you find yourself thinking about the foods that you are not able to eat, you will be heading toward failure.

By now, your cardiovascular system is beginning to improve, and your workouts will begin to get easier. Do not forget that if you can jog longer than the time that is required, do it! The longer you jog, the faster you will get results.

By now you may want to step onto the scale. If you step onto the scale, you will breach the agreement that you made when you began this program, and you will need to start back at the beginning of this program in order to give yourself credit for completing it. That scale is a disaster waiting to happen. If you have a scale, it should be hidden in your house, and under no circumstance should you retrieve it. You will thank me for this when you get on the scale at the end of the program.

Your ketone test strip should indicate a large amount of ketones. If it is still showing only a trace of ketones, you need to monitor your carbohydrate intake more closely.

Make sure that you monitor your breathing and complete every exercise required. You are doing great! Keep going!

Day 6

Date: _____ / _____ / _____

Daily caloric-intake limit: _____ Daily carbohydrate limit: 20

List everything that you need to accomplish today

_____
_____
_____
_____
_____

List the foods that you intend to consume today

_____
_____
_____
_____
_____

List the caloric and carbohydrate totals from the foods you consumed

Food source: _____ Caloric total: _____ Carbohydrate total: ___
Food source: _____ Caloric total: _____ Carbohydrate total: ___
Food source: _____ Caloric total: _____ Carbohydrate total: ___
Food source: _____ Caloric total: _____ Carbohydrate total: ___
Food source: _____ Caloric total: _____ Carbohydrate total: ___
Food source: _____ Caloric total: _____ Carbohydrate total: ___
Food source: _____ Caloric total: _____ Carbohydrate total: ___
Food source: _____ Caloric total: _____ Carbohydrate total: ___
Food source: _____ Caloric total: _____ Carbohydrate total: ___
Food source: _____ Caloric total: _____ Carbohydrate total: ___

Daily caloric total: _____ Daily carbohydrate total: _____

List the amount of time you were able to jog and walk

Jog: _____ Walk: _____

Place a check mark next to your current ketone level

None: _____ Trace: _____ Moderate: _____ Large: _____ High: _____

DAY 7

Self-Discipline
1. Make a list of everything that you need to do today.
2. Maintain the organization of the areas that you most commonly frequent.
3. Do not allow yourself to think about anything that does not support your goals and beliefs.
Diet
1. Make a list of all the foods that you will eat today.
2. List all of the calories and carbohydrates in the meals you consume.
3. Do not exceed your daily caloric and carbohydrate allowance.
Exercise
1. Jog at least 7 minutes, then walk 23 minutes at a fast pace.
2. Start your exercise within the first hour that you are awake.
3. Drink 16 ounces of water before and after your workout.

Daily Expectations

Today will be a very special day for you. You have just successfully completed one week of the most intense fat-loss program ever designed. Only one in twelve individuals ever makes it to this point. I did not let you know that earlier, because I did not want to give your mind any more excuses for not completing this program. Now that you have one week under your belt, you have a 36 percent chance of completing this program in its entirety. That is an awesome statistic.

Remember that if you can complete this entire program, you will be able to maintain a lean body for the remainder of your life. You still do not know the full impact of what you are going to gain over the next twenty-three days.

Today your ketone test strip should indicate a large amount of ketones.

Your energy level is going to be fantastic today. You should feel wonderful after getting through something that most people can only dream about. What you have experienced up to this point is nothing in comparison to what you will experience later in this program. I want you to fully acknowledge the power that is within you. Make sure that you monitor your breathing and complete every exercise required. You are doing better than you know right now. Keep going!

Day 7
Date: _____ / _____ / _____
Daily caloric-intake limit: _____ Daily carbohydrate limit: 20
List everything that you need to accomplish today

_____
_____
_____
_____
_____

List the foods that you intend to consume today

_____
_____
_____
_____
_____

List the caloric and carbohydrate totals from the foods you consumed
Food source: _____ Caloric total: _____ Carbohydrate total: ___
Food source: _____ Caloric total: _____ Carbohydrate total: ___
Food source: _____ Caloric total: _____ Carbohydrate total: ___
Food source: _____ Caloric total: _____ Carbohydrate total: ___
Food source: _____ Caloric total: _____ Carbohydrate total: ___
Food source: _____ Caloric total: _____ Carbohydrate total: ___
Food source: _____ Caloric total: _____ Carbohydrate total: ___
Food source: _____ Caloric total: _____ Carbohydrate total: ___
Food source: _____ Caloric total: _____ Carbohydrate total: ___
Food source: _____ Caloric total: _____ Carbohydrate total: ___
Daily caloric total: _____ Daily carbohydrate total: _____
List the amount of time you were able to jog and walk
Jog: _____ Walk: _____
Place a check mark next to your current ketone level
None: _____ Trace: _____ Moderate: _____ Large: _____ High: _____

DAY 8

Self-Discipline
1. Make a list of everything that you need to do today.
2. Maintain the organization of the areas that you most commonly frequent.
3. Do not allow yourself to think about anything that does not support your goals and beliefs.

Diet
1. Make a list of all the foods that you will eat today.
2. List all of the calories and carbohydrates in the meals you consume.
3. Do not exceed your daily caloric and carbohydrate allowance.

Exercise
1. Jog at least 8 minutes, then walk 22 minutes at a fast pace.
2. Start your exercise within the first hour that you are awake.
3. Drink 16 ounces of water before and after your workout.

Daily Expectations

Today you can expect to feel great! You have already completed the toughest portion of the program. Now you will have to deal with maintaining momentum. This brings on an entirely new challenge. Once you know that you have obtained something, it is a natural reaction to begin to slow down your momentum. The moment you lose even a small amount of momentum, you are heading for disaster. You have to remain extremely focused so that you do not get sidetracked. You need to remember that the first time you begin to take your mind off completing this program, you will change the direction of your focus.

Today you should make an effort to think again about the reasons you wanted to lose the excess body fat in the first place. Every time your mind begins to drift away from your goal, you need to redirect it toward the goal of completing this program.

Today your ketone test strip should still indicate a large amount of ketones.

You may notice that your workout is a little more difficult than what it was yesterday. Now that you have succeeded with your diet, you will need to focus on maintaining momentum with your workouts. Your energy should be fantastic, but you may find that you are beginning to get used to the habit of working out, and you are not quite as excited to complete your workout as you were last week.

Make sure that you monitor your breathing and complete every exercise required. You are doing great. Keep up the good work!

Day 8

Date: _____ / _____ / _____

Daily caloric-intake limit: _____ Daily carbohydrate limit: 20

List everything that you need to accomplish today

_____

_____

_____

_____

_____

List the foods that you intend to consume today

_____

_____

_____

_____

_____

List the caloric and carbohydrate totals from the foods you consumed

Food source: _____ Caloric total: _____ Carbohydrate total: ___

Food source: _____ Caloric total: _____ Carbohydrate total: ___

Food source: _____ Caloric total: _____ Carbohydrate total: ___

Food source: _____ Caloric total: _____ Carbohydrate total: ___

Food source: _____ Caloric total: _____ Carbohydrate total: ___

Food source: _____ Caloric total: _____ Carbohydrate total: ___

Food source: _____ Caloric total: _____ Carbohydrate total: ___

Food source: _____ Caloric total: _____ Carbohydrate total: ___

Food source: _____ Caloric total: _____ Carbohydrate total: ___

Food source: _____ Caloric total: _____ Carbohydrate total: ___

Daily caloric total: _____ Daily carbohydrate total: _____

List the amount of time you were able to jog and walk

Jog: _____ Walk: _____

Place a check mark next to your current ketone level

None: _____ Trace: _____ Moderate: _____ Large: _____ High: _____

DAY 9

Self-Discipline
1. Make a list of everything that you need to do today.
2. Maintain the organization of the areas that you most commonly frequent.
3. Do not allow yourself to think about anything that does not support your goals and beliefs.

Diet
1. Make a list of all the foods that you will eat today.
2. List all of the calories and carbohydrates in the meals you consume.
3. Do not exceed your daily caloric and carbohydrate allowance.

Exercise
1. Jog at least 9 minutes, then walk 21 minutes at a fast pace.
2. Start your exercise within the first hour that you are awake.
3. Drink 16 ounces of water before and after your workout.

Daily Expectations

Today you can expect to feel as if you have things under control. You are beginning to become accustomed to the routine, and you should feel great about your diet. By now your diet will be one of the easiest parts of the program. If you are still experiencing uncomfortable food cravings, you need to pay closer attention to your thoughts. If you are still dealing with cravings, you need to become more aggressive in controlling the thoughts that you allow into your mind. The moment a thought that does not support your eating a low-carbohydrate meal enters your mind, you need to redirect that thought to a low-carbohydrate food. If you are craving pasta, you need to redirect that thought to chicken breast. If you wait any length of time between the first thought and the next, you are opening yourself up to doubt. Once that happens, you will be going the wrong direction. You have been able to come this far because you have remained focused. Keep your mind on the goal of completing this program, and the program will take care of the fat.

Your ketone test strip should still be indicating a large amount of ketones.

Your energy level should be stable, but make sure you do not get complacent in your ability to complete this program. Make sure that you monitor your breathing and complete every exercise required. You have to remain aggressive at all hours of the day. Keep up the good work!

Day 9

Date: _____ / _____ / _____

Daily caloric-intake limit: _____ Daily carbohydrate limit: 20

List everything that you need to accomplish today

_____

_____

_____

_____

_____

List the foods that you intend to consume today

_____

_____

_____

_____

_____

List the caloric and carbohydrate totals from the foods you consumed

Food source: _____ Caloric total: _____ Carbohydrate total: ___

Food source: _____ Caloric total: _____ Carbohydrate total: ___

Food source: _____ Caloric total: _____ Carbohydrate total: ___

Food source: _____ Caloric total: _____ Carbohydrate total: ___

Food source: _____ Caloric total: _____ Carbohydrate total: ___

Food source: _____ Caloric total: _____ Carbohydrate total: ___

Food source: _____ Caloric total: _____ Carbohydrate total: ___

Food source: _____ Caloric total: _____ Carbohydrate total: ___

Food source: _____ Caloric total: _____ Carbohydrate total: ___

Food source: _____ Caloric total: _____ Carbohydrate total: ___

Daily caloric total: _____ Daily carbohydrate total: _____

List the amount of time you were able to jog and walk

Jog: _____ Walk: _____

Place a check mark next to your current ketone level

None: _____ Trace: _____ Moderate: _____ Large: _____ High: _____

DAY 10

Self-Discipline
1. Make a list of everything that you need to do today.
2. Maintain the organization of the areas that you most commonly frequent.
3. Do not allow yourself to think about anything that does not support your goals and beliefs.

Diet
1. Make a list of all the foods that you will eat today.
2. List all of the calories and carbohydrates in the meals you consume.
3. Do not exceed your daily caloric and carbohydrate allowance.

Exercise
1. Jog at least 10 minutes, then walk 20 minutes at a fast pace.
2. Start your exercise within the first hour that you are awake.
3. Drink 16 ounces of water before and after your workout.

Daily Expectations

Today is going to be another stable day. You are going to begin to think things are easy. I am going to warn you: You are not even halfway through, so do not become lazy. At any given time in this program, you could be hit by a craving that will cause you to fail. You have to always be on watch. The moment that you begin to think this program is easy, you will open yourself up for weakness. A craving can come at any given time. If you are not ready to handle it, you could lose everything you have worked so hard for. Do not take this feeling of stability for granted; it can disappear as quickly as it arrived.

Your energy should be stabilized. If you feel tired, it may be a result of not remaining focused. Energy is only a state of mind to pump you up. When you are in the middle of a workout, I want you to really pump yourself up. You can do this by thinking about all of the things that you have accomplished up to this point. Utilize this technique every time you work out. You will be amazed at the energy you can generate with positive thoughts.

Your ketone test strip should still indicate a large amount of ketones.

Make sure that you monitor your breathing and complete every exercise required. Your energy level is going to be great once you pump yourself up with those positive thoughts. Keep going!

Day 10

Date: _____ / _____ / _____

Daily caloric-intake limit: _____ Daily carbohydrate limit: 20

List everything that you need to accomplish today

_____

_____

_____

_____

_____

List the foods that you intend to consume today

_____

_____

_____

_____

_____

List the caloric and carbohydrate totals from the foods you consumed

Food source: _____ Caloric total: _____ Carbohydrate total: ___

Food source: _____ Caloric total: _____ Carbohydrate total: ___

Food source: _____ Caloric total: _____ Carbohydrate total: ___

Food source: _____ Caloric total: _____ Carbohydrate total: ___

Food source: _____ Caloric total: _____ Carbohydrate total: ___

Food source: _____ Caloric total: _____ Carbohydrate total: ___

Food source: _____ Caloric total: _____ Carbohydrate total: ___

Food source: _____ Caloric total: _____ Carbohydrate total: ___

Food source: _____ Caloric total: _____ Carbohydrate total: ___

Food source: _____ Caloric total: _____ Carbohydrate total: ___

Daily caloric total: _____ Daily carbohydrate total: _____

List the amount of time you were able to jog and walk

Jog: _____ Walk: _____

Place a check mark next to your current ketone level

None: _____ Trace: _____ Moderate: _____ Large: _____ High: _____

DAY 11

Self-Discipline
1. Make a list of everything that you need to do today.
2. Maintain the organization of the areas that you most commonly frequent.
3. Do not allow yourself to think about anything that does not support your goals and beliefs.

Diet
1. Make a list of all the foods that you will eat today.
2. List all of the calories and carbohydrates in the meals you consume.
3. Do not exceed your daily caloric and carbohydrate allowance.

Exercise
1. Jog at least 11 minutes, then walk 19 minutes at a fast pace.
2. Start your exercise within the first hour that you are awake.
3. Drink 16 ounces of water before and after your workout.

Daily Expectations

Today you can expect to feel great. Your body has stabilized, and you should have a clear focus on what you expect to gain by completing this program. Today I want you to really focus on jogging as many minutes as possible. If you can jog 15 minutes, do it. I cannot stress enough how much fat your body is burning. The more you exercise, the more fat will be removed from your body. It is a very simple solution, but a very difficult action for some people. You have to begin pushing yourself as hard as you can. You should not have any problems with your diet at this point, so you need to focus on jogging for as long as possible.

Make sure that you are drinking at least sixteen ounces of water before and after your workout. Water will help aid your body in removing the excess body fat. I hope that you are not depriving your body of the proper hydration. If you start to experience signs of dehydration, you know that you need to increase the amount of water that you are consuming.

Your ketone test strip should indicate that you still have a large amount of ketones.

Your energy level should be great, and you can look forward to even more as you go along. Make sure that you monitor your breathing and complete every exercise required. Keep up the good work! You are doing great!

Day 11

Date: _____ / _____ / _____

Daily caloric-intake limit: _____ Daily carbohydrate limit: 20

List everything that you need to accomplish today

_____

_____

_____

_____

_____

List the foods that you intend to consume today

_____

_____

_____

_____

_____

List the caloric and carbohydrate totals from the foods you consumed

Food source: _____ Caloric total: _____ Carbohydrate total: ___

Food source: _____ Caloric total: _____ Carbohydrate total: ___

Food source: _____ Caloric total: _____ Carbohydrate total: ___

Food source: _____ Caloric total: _____ Carbohydrate total: ___

Food source: _____ Caloric total: _____ Carbohydrate total: ___

Food source: _____ Caloric total: _____ Carbohydrate total: ___

Food source: _____ Caloric total: _____ Carbohydrate total: ___

Food source: _____ Caloric total: _____ Carbohydrate total: ___

Food source: _____ Caloric total: _____ Carbohydrate total: ___

Food source: _____ Caloric total: _____ Carbohydrate total: ___

Daily caloric total: _____ Daily carbohydrate total: _____

List the amount of time you were able to jog and walk

Jog: _____ Walk: _____

Place a check mark next to your current ketone level

None: _____ Trace: _____ Moderate: _____ Large: _____ High: _____

DAY 12

Self-Discipline
1. Make a list of everything that you need to do today.
2. Maintain the organization of the areas that you most commonly frequent.
3. Do not allow yourself to think about anything that does not support your goals and beliefs.

Diet
1. Make a list of all the foods that you will eat today.
2. List all of the calories and carbohydrates in the meals you consume.
3. Do not exceed your daily caloric and carbohydrate allowance.

Exercise
1. Jog at least 12 minutes, then walk 18 minutes at a fast pace.
2. Start your exercise within the first hour that you are awake.
3. Drink 16 ounces of water before and after your workout.

Daily Expectations

Today you can expect to feel content. As you get closer to the midway mark, you will begin to enjoy the benefits that go along with conquering your old demons. You are going to notice some of the most dramatic effects of this program within the next couple of weeks.

I am going to focus on your exercise regimen again today. When you are jogging, breath in through your nose and out through your mouth. Focus on your breathing from this point forward. Make sure that you are able to speak at any point in your exercise session. If you are not able to speak while you are jogging, that is a good indication that you are not breathing in enough oxygen. If you are not able to breathe properly, you need to extend the period of time you're walking. Instead of walking eighteen minutes, you need to walk thirty minutes. This will build up your cardiovascular system to a point at which you can breathe normally.

If you feel at any point that you are not able to complete the jogging section of your workout, you need to start over at the beginning of this program. Your body is just not ready for this level of exertion yet. By the time you build your way back up to jogging twelve minutes, you should be able to successfully complete this portion of the program. Nothing comes before your safety.

Your ketone test strip should still indicate a large amount of ketones.

Make sure that you monitor your breathing and complete every exercise required. Your energy level should still be stable, and you can expect it to increase in the days to come. Keep up the good work!

Day 12

Date: _____ / _____ / _____

Daily caloric-intake limit: _____ Daily carbohydrate limit: 20

List everything that you need to accomplish today

_____
_____
_____
_____
_____

List the foods that you intend to consume today

_____
_____
_____
_____
_____

List the caloric and carbohydrate totals from the foods you consumed

Food source: _____ Caloric total: _____ Carbohydrate total: ___
Food source: _____ Caloric total: _____ Carbohydrate total: ___
Food source: _____ Caloric total: _____ Carbohydrate total: ___
Food source: _____ Caloric total: _____ Carbohydrate total: ___
Food source: _____ Caloric total: _____ Carbohydrate total: ___
Food source: _____ Caloric total: _____ Carbohydrate total: ___
Food source: _____ Caloric total: _____ Carbohydrate total: ___
Food source: _____ Caloric total: _____ Carbohydrate total: ___
Food source: _____ Caloric total: _____ Carbohydrate total: ___
Food source: _____ Caloric total: _____ Carbohydrate total: ___

Daily caloric total: _____ Daily carbohydrate total: _____

List the amount of time you were able to jog and walk

Jog: _____ Walk: _____

Place a check mark next to your current ketone level

None: _____ Trace: _____ Moderate: _____ Large: _____ High: _____

DAY 13

Self-Discipline
1. Make a list of everything that you need to do today.
2. Maintain the organization of the areas that you most commonly frequent.
3. Do not allow yourself to think about anything that does not support your goals and beliefs.

Diet
1. Make a list of all the foods that you will eat today.
2. List all of the calories and carbohydrates in the meals you consume.
3. Do not exceed your daily caloric and carbohydrate allowance.

Exercise
1. Jog at least 13 minutes, then walk 17 minutes at a fast pace.
2. Start your exercise within the first hour that you are awake.
3. Drink 16 ounces of water before and after your workout.

Daily Expectations

Today you can expect possibly to be challenged in the area of self-discipline. You will need to really focus on redirecting destructive thoughts. When you know that you are beginning to reach the midway mark of the program, you will begin to feel anxious about completing the program. This anxiety can quickly turn into frustration and will end up destroying all that you have worked for.

Today I want you to focus on observing your internal dialogue. You need to pay close attention to the types of thoughts that you are having. Do your thoughts support your goal of completing this program? Or are your thoughts centered on the things that you are missing out on? This is a potentially danger-ous day for your level of self-discipline, so you need to make an extra effort to be really strong and highly motivated. Once you are able to get through today, you will feel better about your ability to turn up the intensity on maintaining self-dis-cipline.

Your ketone strip should still indicate a large amount of ketones.

Make sure that you monitor your breathing and complete every exercise required. Your energy may be somewhat challenged today, so make that extra effort to stay positive and keep going!

Day 13
Date: _____ / _____ / _____
Daily caloric-intake limit: _____ Daily carbohydrate limit: 20
List everything that you need to accomplish today

_____
_____
_____
_____
_____

List the foods that you intend to consume today

_____
_____
_____
_____
_____

List the caloric and carbohydrate totals from the foods you consumed
Food source: _____ Caloric total: _____ Carbohydrate total: ___
Food source: _____ Caloric total: _____ Carbohydrate total: ___
Food source: _____ Caloric total: _____ Carbohydrate total: ___
Food source: _____ Caloric total: _____ Carbohydrate total: ___
Food source: _____ Caloric total: _____ Carbohydrate total: ___
Food source: _____ Caloric total: _____ Carbohydrate total: ___
Food source: _____ Caloric total: _____ Carbohydrate total: ___
Food source: _____ Caloric total: _____ Carbohydrate total: ___
Food source: _____ Caloric total: _____ Carbohydrate total: ___
Food source: _____ Caloric total: _____ Carbohydrate total: ___
Daily caloric total: _____ Daily carbohydrate total: _____
List the amount of time you were able to jog and walk
Jog: _____ Walk: _____
Place a check mark next to your current ketone level
None: _____ Trace: _____ Moderate: _____ Large: _____ High: _____

DAY 14

Self-Discipline
1. Make a list of everything that you need to do today.
2. Maintain the organization of the areas that you most commonly frequent.
3. Do not allow yourself to think about anything that does not support your goals and beliefs.

Diet
1. Make a list of all the foods that you will eat today.
2. List all of the calories and carbohydrates in the meals you consume.
3. Do not exceed your daily caloric and carbohydrate allowance.

Exercise
1. Jog at least 14 minutes, then walk 16 minutes at a fast pace.
2. Start your exercise within the first hour that you are awake.
3. Drink 16 ounces of water before and after your workout.

Daily Expectations

Today you can expect to feel fantastic. You should have a better understanding of the power that you are beginning to develop. When you have thoughts about things that go against your beliefs and stop those thoughts before they even have a chance to affect your mood, you know that you are beginning to create abilities that you did not previously have. If you were somewhat challenged yesterday, and you utilized the exercise I suggested, you are possibly beginning to understand just how good your future will be.

Happiness is nothing more than a state of mind. When you are able to focus on the things that support what you believe in, your life is going to change dramatically. Now that you have gotten past the first two weeks, your life will begin to look much brighter. Your mind now fully understands the power of your newfound gifts. It is now going to be very difficult for someone to ruin your day, because you can dictate the mood you wish to be in. The good news for you is that it only gets better from here on out.

Your ketone test strip should still indicate that you have a large amount of ketones.

Make sure that you monitor your breathing and complete every exercise required. Your energy level should be absolutely amazing today. Keep up the determination!

Day 14

Date: _____ / _____ / _____

Daily caloric-intake limit: _____ Daily carbohydrate limit: 20

List everything that you need to accomplish today

_____

_____

_____

_____

_____

List the foods that you intend to consume today

_____

_____

_____

_____

_____

List the caloric and carbohydrate totals from the foods you consumed

Food source: _____ Caloric total: _____ Carbohydrate total: ___

Food source: _____ Caloric total: _____ Carbohydrate total: ___

Food source: _____ Caloric total: _____ Carbohydrate total: ___

Food source: _____ Caloric total: _____ Carbohydrate total: ___

Food source: _____ Caloric total: _____ Carbohydrate total: ___

Food source: _____ Caloric total: _____ Carbohydrate total: ___

Food source: _____ Caloric total: _____ Carbohydrate total: ___

Food source: _____ Caloric total: _____ Carbohydrate total: ___

Food source: _____ Caloric total: _____ Carbohydrate total: ___

Food source: _____ Caloric total: _____ Carbohydrate total: ___

Daily caloric total: _____ Daily carbohydrate total: _____

List the amount of time you were able to jog and walk

Jog: _____ Walk: _____

Place a check mark next to your current ketone level

None: _____ Trace: _____ Moderate: _____ Large: _____ High: _____

DAY 15

Self-Discipline
1. Make a list of everything that you need to do today.
2. Maintain the organization of the areas that you most commonly frequent.
3. Do not allow yourself to think about anything that does not support your goals and beliefs.

Diet
1. Make a list of all the foods that you will eat today.
2. List all of the calories and carbohydrates in the meals you consume.
3. Do not exceed your daily caloric and carbohydrate allowance.

Exercise
1. Jog at least 15 minutes, then walk 15 minutes at a fast pace.
2. Start your exercise within the first hour that you are awake.
3. Drink 16 ounces of water before and after your workout.

Daily Expectations

Today you can expect to feel more confident than you ever have at any point in your life. You have just completed half of the entire program. You now have a 62 percent chance of completing the program. I cannot stress enough how impressed I am with you at this point. To make it this far into the program, you have to be one dedicated individual. As with anyone who completes this program, I would love to meet you at some point, because you truly are one in about a thousand people, one who has the guts to strengthen your own character.

From this point forward, I will focus on some of the most powerful techniques available in order to take your new strengths to the next level. You deserve everything that you have coming to you over the next couple of weeks. It is my pleasure to share with you some of the most powerful techniques available to increase your confidence, self-esteem, and self-discipline. Anyone who can endure what you have up to this point deserves to live the best life possible. Enjoy your success today, because we are going to turn up the intensity tomorrow. Congratulations—you have absolutely proven your inner strength.

Your ketone test strip should still show a large amount of ketones.

Make sure that you monitor your breathing and complete every exercise required. Your energy level will be uncontainable today. You are now jogging for at least fifteen minutes. That is fantastic! Keep up the good work!

Day 15

Date: _____ / _____ / _____

Daily caloric-intake limit: _____ Daily carbohydrate limit: 20

List everything that you need to accomplish today

_____

_____

_____

_____

_____

List the foods that you intend to consume today

_____

_____

_____

_____

_____

List the caloric and carbohydrate totals from the foods you consumed

Food source: _____ Caloric total: _____ Carbohydrate total: ___

Food source: _____ Caloric total: _____ Carbohydrate total: ___

Food source: _____ Caloric total: _____ Carbohydrate total: ___

Food source: _____ Caloric total: _____ Carbohydrate total: ___

Food source: _____ Caloric total: _____ Carbohydrate total: ___

Food source: _____ Caloric total: _____ Carbohydrate total: ___

Food source: _____ Caloric total: _____ Carbohydrate total: ___

Food source: _____ Caloric total: _____ Carbohydrate total: ___

Food source: _____ Caloric total: _____ Carbohydrate total: ___

Food source: _____ Caloric total: _____ Carbohydrate total: ___

Daily caloric total: _____ Daily carbohydrate total: _____

List the amount of time you were able to jog and walk

Jog: _____ Walk: _____

Place a check mark next to your current ketone level

None: _____ Trace: _____ Moderate: _____ Large: _____ High: _____

DAY 16

Self-Discipline
1. Make a list of everything that you need to do today.
2. Maintain the organization of the areas that you most commonly frequent.
3. Do not allow yourself to think about anything that does not support your goals and beliefs.

Diet
1. Make a list of all the foods that you will eat today.
2. List all of the calories and carbohydrates in the meals you consume.
3. Do not exceed your daily caloric and carbohydrate allowance.

Exercise
1. Jog at least 16 minutes, then walk 14 minutes at a fast pace.
2. Start your exercise within the first hour that you are awake.
3. Drink 16 ounces of water before and after your workout.

Daily Expectations

Today you can expect to feel very confident. But I urge you to remain balanced. If you become too excited about getting the first half of the program under your belt, you may get off balance and lose control. Now that you are beginning to realize that you have more self-control than you may have believed possible, it is time to begin enhancing that ability.

First I want you to begin controlling your emotions, which is much more difficult than most people would like to believe. In order to control your emotions, you must utilize the self-discipline that you are beginning to establish. The moment you get an urge to do something that you know goes against your goals and beliefs, back off and just relax. The ability to relax when the rest of the world is knocking on your door is very difficult at times. This is when your breathing exercises are going to really show their effectiveness.

We are going to start with your stored memories and work our way out to other peoples' actions. Today I want you to remember one incident in your past when you felt like you were losing control of your life. Everyone has had this experience at least once in their lives. Now that you have that image in your head, relax instead of having a reaction to that memory. Just relax. This one memory is the only thing I want you to think about today. I want you to keep replaying that memory until you are able to recall that memory without any reaction or emotion. Remain patient, because this may take some time; do not overlook this exercise. This exercise will set up the remainder of this program. Stay focused!

Your ketone test strip should still indicate a large amount of ketones.

Make sure that you monitor your breathing and complete every exercise required. Today is going to be a very mental day, so stay calm and you will do just fine!

Day 16

Date: _____ / _____ / _____

Daily caloric-intake limit: _____ Daily carbohydrate limit: 20

List everything that you need to accomplish today

_____
_____
_____
_____
_____

List the foods that you intend to consume today

_____
_____
_____
_____
_____

List the caloric and carbohydrate totals from the foods you consumed

Food source: _____ Caloric total: _____ Carbohydrate total: ___
Food source: _____ Caloric total: _____ Carbohydrate total: ___
Food source: _____ Caloric total: _____ Carbohydrate total: ___
Food source: _____ Caloric total: _____ Carbohydrate total: ___
Food source: _____ Caloric total: _____ Carbohydrate total: ___
Food source: _____ Caloric total: _____ Carbohydrate total: ___
Food source: _____ Caloric total: _____ Carbohydrate total: ___
Food source: _____ Caloric total: _____ Carbohydrate total: ___
Food source: _____ Caloric total: _____ Carbohydrate total: ___
Food source: _____ Caloric total: _____ Carbohydrate total: ___

Daily caloric total: _____ Daily carbohydrate total: _____

List the amount of time you were able to jog and walk

Jog: _____Walk: _____

Place a check mark next to your current ketone level

None: _____ Trace: _____ Moderate: _____ Large: _____ High: _____

DAY 17

Self-Discipline
1. Make a list of everything that you need to do today.
2. Maintain the organization of the areas that you most commonly frequent.
3. Do not allow yourself to think about anything that does not support your goals and beliefs.

Diet
1. Make a list of all the foods that you will eat today.
2. List all of the calories and carbohydrates in the meals you consume.
3. Do not exceed your daily caloric and carbohydrate allowance.

Exercise
1. Jog at least 17 minutes, then walk 13 minutes at a fast pace.
2. Start your exercise within the first hour that you are awake.
3. Drink 16 ounces of water before and after your workout.

Daily Expectations

Today you may feel somewhat frustrated. The lesson you completed yesterday is not always easy. To recall an uncomfortable feeling that is attached to a harmful memory can often be an unpleasant experience. I hope that you remained focused and accomplished the task of conquering that one memory.

Today we will move on to another memory. I want you to recall another unpleasant memory and stay calm once again. You may have already moved on to other memories after experiencing the power of this exercise. The ability to control your emotions is without question the most powerful ability you will ever possess. When you reach a level at which no one can say or do anything to throw you off balance, you will have reached a place of absolute certainty. You will no longer be controlled by the people around you, and you will be able to remain focused on the things you want in life. I want you to continue to keep replaying your memories until you have successfully cleaned up all of the baggage from your past. This process happens much faster than one may think. You have the ability to clean up a lifetime of pain and hurt in the matter of days. I hope that you will take this exercise seriously, because your life will never be the same once you reestablish control over your thoughts and emotions.

Your ketone test strip should still indicate a large amount of ketones.

Make sure that you monitor your breathing and complete every exercise required. Your energy level should feel stabilized. It can sometimes be very strenuous work when you deal with exercises of the mind. Take your time, and you will begin to see rather quickly just how close you are not only to losing all of your excess body fat, but to keeping it off for life. Keep up the intensity!

Day 17

Date: _____ / _____ / _____

Daily caloric-intake limit: _____ Daily carbohydrate limit: 20

List everything that you need to accomplish today

_____
_____
_____
_____
_____

List the foods that you intend to consume today

_____
_____
_____
_____
_____

List the caloric and carbohydrate totals from the foods you consumed

Food source: _____ Caloric total: _____ Carbohydrate total: ___
Food source: _____ Caloric total: _____ Carbohydrate total: ___
Food source: _____ Caloric total: _____ Carbohydrate total: ___
Food source: _____ Caloric total: _____ Carbohydrate total: ___
Food source: _____ Caloric total: _____ Carbohydrate total: ___
Food source: _____ Caloric total: _____ Carbohydrate total: ___
Food source: _____ Caloric total: _____ Carbohydrate total: ___
Food source: _____ Caloric total: _____ Carbohydrate total: ___
Food source: _____ Caloric total: _____ Carbohydrate total: ___
Food source: _____ Caloric total: _____ Carbohydrate total: ___

Daily caloric total: _____ Daily carbohydrate total: _____

List the amount of time you were able to jog and walk

Jog: _____ Walk: _____

Place a check mark next to your current ketone level

None: _____ Trace: _____ Moderate: _____ Large: _____ High: _____

DAY 18

Self-Discipline

1. Make a list of everything that you need to do today.
2. Maintain the organization of the areas that you most commonly frequent.
3. Do not allow yourself to think about anything that does not support your goals and beliefs.

Diet

1. Make a list of all the foods that you will eat today.
2. List all of the calories and carbohydrates in the meals you consume.
3. Do not exceed your daily caloric and carbohydrate allowance.

Exercise

1. Jog at least 18 minutes, then walk 12 minutes at a fast pace.
2. Start your exercise within the first hour that you are awake.
3. Drink 16 ounces of water before and after your workout.

Daily Expectations

Today you may feel somewhat focused. As you continue to clean up the painful experiences from your past, you will begin to focus more on the things that bring you pleasure. I want you to take the time to really understand the topic that I am preparing to discuss.

When you find something that upsets you or causes you to have a negative reaction, that memory will seem louder than the memories that bring you pleasure. If you were scared of something as a child, that memory will have a strong feeling attached to it. The level of fear you experienced will determine the amount of feeling that you have attached to that memory.

The secret to maintaining self-discipline is always to be centered. In order to do this, you have to be able to control your reactions to the world around you. This is not accomplished in one day, and it will occasionally take people years to accomplish. The ability to control your emotions under all circumstances is possible, and if you remain focused, you will gain this ability in a very short period of time. If you have been taking the previous exercises seriously, you are beginning to understand that you do have control over the things that influence and shape your life. Instead of being controlled by the world around you, you are now in control of your own personal world. The ability that you are now beginning to strengthen is the deepest level of self-discipline.

If you are still dealing with past memories, continue to clean house, but also begin thinking in present time. Think about the reactions you have to the world around you.

Did someone say or do something to you that may have upset you? Start recognizing the impact other people's actions have on your life. Remain focused, as there is a beautiful reaction happening inside of you right now. Just keep going. You will see and feel the results in the following days.

Your ketone strip should still indicate a large amount of ketones.

Make sure that you monitor your breathing and complete every exercise required. Keep going!

Day 18

Date: _____ / _____ / _____

Daily caloric-intake limit: _____ Daily carbohydrate limit: 20

List everything that you need to accomplish today

_____

_____

_____

_____

_____

List the foods that you intend to consume today

_____

_____

_____

_____

_____

List the caloric and carbohydrate totals from the foods you consumed

Food source: _____ Caloric total: _____ Carbohydrate total: ___

Food source: _____ Caloric total: _____ Carbohydrate total: ___

Food source: _____ Caloric total: _____ Carbohydrate total: ___

Food source: _____ Caloric total: _____ Carbohydrate total: ___

Food source: _____ Caloric total: _____ Carbohydrate total: ___

Food source: _____ Caloric total: _____ Carbohydrate total: ___

Food source: _____ Caloric total: _____ Carbohydrate total: ___

Food source: _____ Caloric total: _____ Carbohydrate total: ___

Food source: _____ Caloric total: _____ Carbohydrate total: ___

Food source: _____ Caloric total: _____ Carbohydrate total: ___

Daily caloric total: _____ Daily carbohydrate total: _____

List the amount of time you were able to jog and walk

Jog: _____ Walk: _____

Place a check mark next to your current ketone level

None: _____ Trace: _____ Moderate: _____ Large: _____ High: _____

DAY 19

Self-Discipline
1. Make a list of everything that you need to do today.
2. Maintain the organization of the areas that you most commonly frequent.
3. Do not allow yourself to think about anything that does not support your goals and beliefs.

Diet
1. Make a list of all the foods that you will eat today.
2. List all of the calories and carbohydrates in the meals you consume.
3. Do not exceed your daily caloric and carbohydrate allowance.

Exercise
1. Jog at least 19 minutes, then walk 11 minutes at a fast pace.
2. Start your exercise within the first hour that you are awake.
3. Drink 16 ounces of water before and after your workout.

Daily Expectations

Today you will begin to feel an amazing peace that you may have never felt before. I want you to make sure that the new abilities you gained are always protected and maintained. You are beginning to develop some of the most powerful abilities available to maintain strength and peace of mind.

You will begin to notice some major shifts in your life. The things that once limited you are now creating more strength. The more adversity you face, the stronger you become. I know that you may have heard the saying, "What does not kill you will make you stronger." I agree with that saying, because I have experienced it firsthand. Once I knew that I had the ability to control my emotions, I began to look for tough circumstances to pull myself through. The problem was that I could no longer find tough circumstances, because my mind no longer considered adversity as a difficulty to overcome. I began to look at adversity as a challenge that could easily be overcome, and as a result of that, I continued to become stronger.

I hope that you will begin to experience these types of circumstances in your life as well. I want you to continue with these self-control exercises, as they will become a permanent part of your life. Once you are able to experience the pleasure that comes along with peace, you will begin to crave it. Once that happens, it will be easy for you to remain focused on being centered.

Your ketone test strip should still indicate a large amount of ketones.

Make sure that you monitor your breathing and complete every exercise required. Keep that determination going. You are doing great!

Day 19

Date: _____ / _____ / _____

Daily caloric-intake limit: _____ Daily carbohydrate limit: 20

List everything that you need to accomplish today

_____
_____
_____
_____
_____

List the foods that you intend to consume today

_____
_____
_____
_____
_____

List the caloric and carbohydrate totals from the foods you consumed

Food source: _____ Caloric total: _____ Carbohydrate total: ___
Food source: _____ Caloric total: _____ Carbohydrate total: ___
Food source: _____ Caloric total: _____ Carbohydrate total: ___
Food source: _____ Caloric total: _____ Carbohydrate total: ___
Food source: _____ Caloric total: _____ Carbohydrate total: ___
Food source: _____ Caloric total: _____ Carbohydrate total: ___
Food source: _____ Caloric total: _____ Carbohydrate total: ___
Food source: _____ Caloric total: _____ Carbohydrate total: ___
Food source: _____ Caloric total: _____ Carbohydrate total: ___
Food source: _____ Caloric total: _____ Carbohydrate total: ___

Daily caloric total: _____ Daily carbohydrate total: _____

List the amount of time you were able to jog and walk

Jog: _____Walk: _____

Place a check mark next to your current ketone level

None: _____ Trace: _____ Moderate: _____ Large: _____ High: _____

DAY 20

Self-Discipline
1. Make a list of everything that you need to do today.
2. Maintain the organization of the areas that you most commonly frequent.
3. Do not allow yourself to think about anything that does not support your goals and beliefs.

Diet
1. Make a list of all the foods that you will eat today.
2. List all of the calories and carbohydrates in the meals you consume.
3. Do not exceed your daily caloric and carbohydrate allowance.

Exercise
1. Jog at least 20 minutes, then walk 10 minutes at a fast pace.
2. Start your exercise within the first hour that you are awake.
3. Drink 16 ounces of water before and after your workout.

Daily Expectations

Today will be a great day. You are beginning to develop the abilities that I promised you in the beginning of this program. The feeling that you have is a direct result of your determination to get what you have always wanted in life. When you combine self-discipline with a diet and exercise program, you have a formula that provides physical proof that you do have control over your behavior. You are beginning to realize that you have this ability, and there is a lot of peace that comes along with it. I do not want you to stop there. Trust me; I have trained thousands of clients who began to experience the benefits that come along with strong self-discipline. The stronger you become, the more benefits you will receive. The pleasure and peace that you are beginning to experience is just a start. I promise you that they will continue to increase over time.

The most common mistake I see people make is that they see the finish line and begin to weaken. I do not know if you have ever watched a triathlon, but many times, a runner will collapse just prior to reaching the finish line. The moment you begin to reduce your intensity is the moment you become stagnant. Self-control is a constant work in progress. It never stops; you will be maintaining self-discipline until the day you die. The moment you give up is the moment that you die. I urge you to keep pushing yourself. Do not become content with your newfound abilities. They will only get better.

Your ketone test strips should still indicate a large amount of ketones.

Make sure that you monitor your breathing and complete every exercise required. Stay focused and keep up the intensity!

Day 20

Date: _____ / _____ / _____

Daily caloric-intake limit: _____ Daily carbohydrate limit: 20

List everything that you need to accomplish today

_____

_____

_____

_____

_____

List the foods that you intend to consume today

_____

_____

_____

_____

_____

List the caloric and carbohydrate totals from the foods you consumed

Food source: _____ Caloric total: _____ Carbohydrate total: ___

Food source: _____ Caloric total: _____ Carbohydrate total: ___

Food source: _____ Caloric total: _____ Carbohydrate total: ___

Food source: _____ Caloric total: _____ Carbohydrate total: ___

Food source: _____ Caloric total: _____ Carbohydrate total: ___

Food source: _____ Caloric total: _____ Carbohydrate total: ___

Food source: _____ Caloric total: _____ Carbohydrate total: ___

Food source: _____ Caloric total: _____ Carbohydrate total: ___

Food source: _____ Caloric total: _____ Carbohydrate total: ___

Food source: _____ Caloric total: _____ Carbohydrate total: ___

Daily caloric total: _____ Daily carbohydrate total: _____

List the amount of time you were able to jog and walk

Jog: _____ Walk: _____

Place a check mark next to your current ketone level

None: _____ Trace: _____ Moderate: _____ Large: _____ High: _____

DAY 21

Self-Discipline
1. Make a list of everything that you need to do today.
2. Maintain the organization of the areas that you most commonly frequent.
3. Do not allow yourself to think about anything that does not support your goals and beliefs.
Diet
1. Make a list of all the foods that you will eat today.
2. List all of the calories and carbohydrates in the meals you consume.
3. Do not exceed your daily caloric and carbohydrate allowance.
Exercise
1. Jog at least 21 minutes, then walk 9 minutes at a fast pace.
2. Start your exercise within the first hour that you are awake.
3. Drink 16 ounces of water before and after your workout.

Daily Expectations

Today you may notice a very strong sense of certainty. This feeling is, without question, the key to happiness. I do not know of another feeling that allows you to maintain a consistent state of joy. The problems that you once struggled with are now beginning to seem weak and distant. The things that would have normally upset you and caused you to react negatively will begin to diminish altogether.

Today I want you only to enjoy this feeling. Be fully aware of the peace you are experiencing as a result of your hard work. You have come a long way over the past three weeks. Every day you have been challenging yourself to succeed. If you have followed every exercise in this program, you now have a deeper understanding of what peace truly is.

Today you should be focused on enjoying your new abilities. Really observe the changes that you have gone through up to this point. Not many individuals will ever get the opportunity to experience this. You are one in a million, one who has the ability to control yourself in all situations. You will be able to choose what you want to think about instead of being compelled to dwell on memories that seek only to harm you.

Even though I have been focused for the past week on self-discipline, I want you to make sure that you are completing your workouts in their entirety. You should be jogging for at least twenty-one minutes. That is fantastic! Not only are you developing a powerful mind, you are creating a powerful body.

Your ketone test strips should still indicate a large amount of ketones.

Make sure that you monitor your breathing and complete every exercise required. Enjoy today, because tomorrow, we will crank up the intensity once again.

Day 21

Date: _____ / _____ / _____

Daily caloric-intake limit: _____ Daily carbohydrate limit: 20

List everything that you need to accomplish today

_____
_____
_____
_____
_____

List the foods that you intend to consume today

_____
_____
_____
_____
_____

List the caloric and carbohydrate totals from the foods you consumed

Food source: _____ Caloric total: _____ Carbohydrate total: ___
Food source: _____ Caloric total: _____ Carbohydrate total: ___
Food source: _____ Caloric total: _____ Carbohydrate total: ___
Food source: _____ Caloric total: _____ Carbohydrate total: ___
Food source: _____ Caloric total: _____ Carbohydrate total: ___
Food source: _____ Caloric total: _____ Carbohydrate total: ___
Food source: _____ Caloric total: _____ Carbohydrate total: ___
Food source: _____ Caloric total: _____ Carbohydrate total: ___
Food source: _____ Caloric total: _____ Carbohydrate total: ___
Food source: _____ Caloric total: _____ Carbohydrate total: ___

Daily caloric total: _____ Daily carbohydrate total: _____

List the amount of time you were able to jog and walk

Jog: _____ Walk: _____

Place a check mark next to your current ketone level

None: _____ Trace: _____ Moderate: _____ Large: _____ High: _____

DAY 22

Self-Discipline
1. Make a list of everything that you need to do today.
2. Maintain the organization of the areas that you most commonly frequent.
3. Do not allow yourself to think about anything that does not support your goals and beliefs.

Diet
1. Make a list of all the foods that you will eat today.
2. List all of the calories and carbohydrates in the meals you consume.
3. Do not exceed your daily caloric and carbohydrate allowance.

Exercise
1. Jog at least 22 minutes, then walk 8 minutes at a fast pace.
2. Start your exercise within the first hour that you are awake.
3. Drink 16 ounces of water before and after your workout.

Daily Expectations

Today you can expect to feel great. You should be so focused by now that you know you are going to complete this program with ease. But I warn you that you are still eight days away from the successful completion of this program.

You have to be jogging at least twenty-two minutes. If you are not able to jog twenty-two minutes, you will need to start over at the beginning of this program. In order to gain the abilities that are offered with this program, you must be able to complete every exercise in this program. No exercise can be overlooked. I urge you to concentrate on your ability to stay focused.

There is no way you could have reached this point in the program if you were not able to take responsibility for your actions. No one who has the heart to reach this far will allow himself or herself to quit. Stay focused and utilize your new abilities to remain disciplined and push yourself to the next level. Make sure that you remain focused on the mental aspects of self-discipline.

Your ketone test strip should still indicate a large amount of ketones.

Make sure that you monitor your breathing and complete every exercise required. Your energy level should be high today. Really focus on your workout today. Make sure that you are jogging the entire twenty-two minutes. Keep going. You are doing great!

Day 22

Date: _____ / _____ / _____

Daily caloric-intake limit: _____ Daily carbohydrate limit: 20

List everything that you need to accomplish today

_____

_____

_____

_____

_____

List the foods that you intend to consume today

_____

_____

_____

_____

_____

List the caloric and carbohydrate totals from the foods you consumed

Food source: _____ Caloric total: _____ Carbohydrate total: ___

Food source: _____ Caloric total: _____ Carbohydrate total: ___

Food source: _____ Caloric total: _____ Carbohydrate total: ___

Food source: _____ Caloric total: _____ Carbohydrate total: ___

Food source: _____ Caloric total: _____ Carbohydrate total: ___

Food source: _____ Caloric total: _____ Carbohydrate total: ___

Food source: _____ Caloric total: _____ Carbohydrate total: ___

Food source: _____ Caloric total: _____ Carbohydrate total: ___

Food source: _____ Caloric total: _____ Carbohydrate total: ___

Food source: _____ Caloric total: _____ Carbohydrate total: ___

Daily caloric total: _____ Daily carbohydrate total: _____

List the amount of time you were able to jog and walk

Jog: _____ Walk: _____

Place a check mark next to your current ketone level

None: _____ Trace: _____ Moderate: _____ Large: _____ High: _____

Day 23

Self-Discipline
1. Make a list of everything that you need to do today.
2. Maintain the organization of the areas that you most commonly frequent.
3. Do not allow yourself to think about anything that does not support your goals and beliefs.

Diet
1. Make a list of all the foods that you will eat today.
2. List all of the calories and carbohydrates in the meals you consume.
3. Do not exceed your daily caloric and carbohydrate allowance.

Exercise
1. Jog at least 23 minutes, then walk 7 minutes at a fast pace.
2. Start your exercise within the first hour that you are awake.
3. Drink 16 ounces of water before and after your workout.

Daily Expectations

Today is truly going to be a special day for you. I have witnessed the majority of my clients finding that at the three-week point, they were able to completely defeat the addiction to food. By now, your addiction to food should be completely defeated. That is a major accomplishment in your fight against body fat. Now that you have defeated your fight against food cravings, you need to make sure that you do not develop an addiction toward something else. I hope that you have been spending a lot of time focusing on strengthening all the areas of your life, not just your addiction to food. I have had some clients who did not complete their self-discipline exercises and experienced a compulsion to develop another habit. This only happened with the clients who did not focus on their self-discipline exercises.

If you have skipped over the self-discipline exercises, you have not completed twenty-three days of this program. Even though you have temporarily defeated your addiction to food, it will come back at some point in your future. The only way you will maintain the results you have achieved up to this point is to focus on maintaining the parameters that surround your beliefs and goals. Utilize this week to really focus on enjoying the certainty that comes along with having intense self-confidence.

I want you to begin utilizing some of the energy you have been conserving. By now, you should have an amazing amount of self-control. Start utilizing it; you have earned it. Accomplish something today that you have been putting off. Begin taking aggressive actions toward accomplishing your goals. Become aggressive and remain focused! You are only a week away from completion.

Your ketone test strip should still indicate a large amount of ketones.

Make sure that you monitor your breathing and complete every exercise required. Your energy level will be high today, because you make it high! Get tough and jog twenty-three minutes!

Day 23

Date: _____ / _____ / _____

Daily caloric-intake limit: _____ Daily carbohydrate limit: 20

List everything that you need to accomplish today

_____
_____
_____
_____
_____

List the foods that you intend to consume today

_____
_____
_____
_____
_____

List the caloric and carbohydrate totals from the foods you consumed

Food source: _____ Caloric total: _____ Carbohydrate total: ___
Food source: _____ Caloric total: _____ Carbohydrate total: ___
Food source: _____ Caloric total: _____ Carbohydrate total: ___
Food source: _____ Caloric total: _____ Carbohydrate total: ___
Food source: _____ Caloric total: _____ Carbohydrate total: ___
Food source: _____ Caloric total: _____ Carbohydrate total: ___
Food source: _____ Caloric total: _____ Carbohydrate total: ___
Food source: _____ Caloric total: _____ Carbohydrate total: ___
Food source: _____ Caloric total: _____ Carbohydrate total: ___
Food source: _____ Caloric total: _____ Carbohydrate total: ___

Daily caloric total: _____ Daily carbohydrate total: _____

List the amount of time you were able to jog and walk

Jog: _____ Walk: _____

Place a check mark next to your current ketone level

None: _____ Trace: _____ Moderate: _____ Large: _____ High: _____

DAY 24

Self-Discipline
1. Make a list of everything that you need to do today.
2. Maintain the organization of the areas that you most commonly frequent.
3. Do not allow yourself to think about anything that does not support your goals and beliefs.

Diet
1. Make a list of all the foods that you will eat today.
2. List all of the calories and carbohydrates in the meals you consume.
3. Do not exceed your daily caloric and carbohydrate allowance.

Exercise
1. Jog at least 24 minutes, then walk 6 minutes at a fast pace.
2. Start your exercise within the first hour that you are awake.
3. Drink 16 ounces of water before and after your workout.

Daily Expectations

Today you should be feeling very comfortable with your ability to remain focused. You are less than a week away from completing one of the most intense fat-loss programs ever designed. You should be developing your own self-discipline exercises by now. You should be developing your own beliefs about how you control your emotions. You are the only one who knows you. Everyone else sees only the image of who you are. You know who you are deep down inside. This ability to know yourself on a deeper level is what will keep you focused once you complete this program. You should be developing a true look at who you are. If you want to be confident, you should be confident. If you want to be strong, you should be strong. The person you are leaving behind is the person who you had to be because you lacked the discipline to take control of your actions.

By now, you should be able to aggressively take full control of your thoughts and actions. You should be starting to understand the importance of letting things go when they begin to frustrate you. When someone says something that upsets you, you should be able to deflect those comments right away. I hope you are developing a deep sense of self. Once you have that, no one can take that away from you.

Your ketone test strip should still indicate a large amount of ketones.

Make sure that you monitor your breathing and complete every exercise required. Stay aggressive. You are only six days away from completing this program!

Day 24

Date: _____ / _____ / _____

Daily caloric-intake limit: _____ Daily carbohydrate limit: 20

List everything that you need to accomplish today

_____
_____
_____
_____
_____

List the foods that you intend to consume today

_____
_____
_____
_____
_____

List the caloric and carbohydrate totals from the foods you consumed

Food source: _____ Caloric total: _____ Carbohydrate total: ___
Food source: _____ Caloric total: _____ Carbohydrate total: ___
Food source: _____ Caloric total: _____ Carbohydrate total: ___
Food source: _____ Caloric total: _____ Carbohydrate total: ___
Food source: _____ Caloric total: _____ Carbohydrate total: ___
Food source: _____ Caloric total: _____ Carbohydrate total: ___
Food source: _____ Caloric total: _____ Carbohydrate total: ___
Food source: _____ Caloric total: _____ Carbohydrate total: ___
Food source: _____ Caloric total: _____ Carbohydrate total: ___
Food source: _____ Caloric total: _____ Carbohydrate total: ___

Daily caloric total: _____ Daily carbohydrate total: _____

List the amount of time you were able to jog and walk

Jog: _____ Walk: _____

Place a check mark next to your current ketone level

None: _____ Trace: _____ Moderate: _____ Large: _____ High: _____

DAY 25

Self-Discipline
1. Make a list of everything that you need to do today.
2. Maintain the organization of the areas that you most commonly frequent.
3. Do not allow yourself to think about anything that does not support your goals and beliefs.
Diet
1. Make a list of all the foods that you will eat today.
2. List all of the calories and carbohydrates in the meals you consume.
3. Do not exceed your daily caloric and carbohydrate allowance.
Exercise
1. Jog at least 25 minutes, then walk 5 minutes at a fast pace.
2. Start your exercise within the first hour that you are awake.
3. Drink 16 ounces of water before and after your workout.

Daily Expectations

Today you will be tempted to begin to relax. I am going to warn you ahead of time: I have seen more clients drop out of this program with five days remaining than you may imagine. You will begin to feel confident in your ability to control your actions. At midnight, you will get up, walk to your refrigerator, and retrieve something out of the refrigerator that you know you shouldn't have.

You have to stay more focused these last few days than you have at any other point in the program. You are close, but you have to be completely focused. You did not come this far to lose it all now. I know that you are enjoying the benefits that come along with intense self-discipline, but you have to be on guard always. A craving can creep up on you at any time. Even though you have completed twenty-five days of extreme fat loss, you still have to remember the tools that brought you here. Every exercise that you have consistently completed through-out this program has brought you to where you are at today. The three funda-mental exercises that you should be doing automatically by now are responsible for your ability to establish, strengthen, and maintain self-discipline. If you had not taken those exercises seriously, you would not have the amazing level of con-fidence that you radiate today. Enjoy your new abilities, but I warn you to remain focused.

Your ketone test strips should still indicate a large amount of ketones.

Make sure that you monitor your breathing and complete every exercise required. Your energy is going to be stabilized because you are focused. Keep going! You are almost there!

Day 25

Date: _____ / _____ / _____

Daily caloric-intake limit: _____ Daily carbohydrate limit: 20

List everything that you need to accomplish today

_____

_____

_____

_____

_____

List the foods that you intend to consume today

_____

_____

_____

_____

_____

List the caloric and carbohydrate totals from the foods you consumed

Food source: _____ Caloric total: _____ Carbohydrate total: ___
Food source: _____ Caloric total: _____ Carbohydrate total: ___
Food source: _____ Caloric total: _____ Carbohydrate total: ___
Food source: _____ Caloric total: _____ Carbohydrate total: ___
Food source: _____ Caloric total: _____ Carbohydrate total: ___
Food source: _____ Caloric total: _____ Carbohydrate total: ___
Food source: _____ Caloric total: _____ Carbohydrate total: ___
Food source: _____ Caloric total: _____ Carbohydrate total: ___
Food source: _____ Caloric total: _____ Carbohydrate total: ___
Food source: _____ Caloric total: _____ Carbohydrate total: ___

Daily caloric total: _____ Daily carbohydrate total: _____

List the amount of time you were able to jog and walk

Jog: _____ Walk: _____

Place a check mark next to your current ketone level

None: _____ Trace: _____ Moderate: _____ Large: _____ High: _____

DAY 26

Self-Discipline
1. Make a list of everything that you need to do today.
2. Maintain the organization of the areas that you most commonly frequent.
3. Do not allow yourself to think about anything that does not support your goals and beliefs.

Diet
1. Make a list of all the foods that you will eat today.
2. List all of the calories and carbohydrates in the meals you consume.
3. Do not exceed your daily caloric and carbohydrate allowance.

Exercise
1. Jog at least 26 minutes, then walk 4 minutes at a fast pace.
2. Start your exercise within the first hour that you are awake.
3. Drink 16 ounces of water before and after your workout.

Daily Expectations

Today you can expect to feel absolutely amazing. You should be exploding with confidence and energy. Nothing can hold you back at this point. I know you have been focusing on staying balanced, but it is time to turn up the intensity. I want you to begin taking aggressive actions toward the things that you have always wanted in life. If you have always wanted to be wealthy, take an aggressive action toward making it happen. You have everything you have ever needed inside of you right now. You have to slowly crank up the intensity. If you are feeling anxious over taking aggressive actions toward completing a goal that you have been putting off, slow down and stay in balance. Move only as fast as you can while staying balanced.

Anything you do from this point on in your life should be balanced. If you begin to feel that you are losing control, just slow down and relax. You will quickly regain the control that you have worked so hard to obtain. You will be able to move only as fast as time will allow. You need to stay focused, but you also need to keep moving ahead. This requires assertive action, with intensity and balance. That is the challenge that you will face for the remainder of your life. The ability to aggressively move toward your goal and still remain focused and centered is the same ability that will allow you to accomplish anything that you want in life. You need to begin polishing your abilities. The finesse that you begin to apply will be responsible for the dramatic effects that you are going to experience.

This ability is possible, and thousands of my clients are already experiencing it daily.

Your ketone test strips should still indicate a large amount of ketones. Make sure that you monitor your breathing and complete every exercise required. Stay focused, but be aggressive!

Day 26

Date: _____ / _____ / _____

Daily caloric-intake limit: _____ Daily carbohydrate limit: 20

List everything that you need to accomplish today

_____
_____
_____
_____
_____

List the foods that you intend to consume today

_____
_____
_____
_____
_____

List the caloric and carbohydrate totals from the foods you consumed

Food source: _____ Caloric total: _____ Carbohydrate total: ___
Food source: _____ Caloric total: _____ Carbohydrate total: ___
Food source: _____ Caloric total: _____ Carbohydrate total: ___
Food source: _____ Caloric total: _____ Carbohydrate total: ___
Food source: _____ Caloric total: _____ Carbohydrate total: ___
Food source: _____ Caloric total: _____ Carbohydrate total: ___
Food source: _____ Caloric total: _____ Carbohydrate total: ___
Food source: _____ Caloric total: _____ Carbohydrate total: ___
Food source: _____ Caloric total: _____ Carbohydrate total: ___
Food source: _____ Caloric total: _____ Carbohydrate total: ___

Daily caloric total: _____ Daily carbohydrate total: _____

List the amount of time you were able to jog and walk

Jog: _____ Walk: _____

Place a check mark next to your current ketone level

None: _____ Trace: _____ Moderate: _____ Large: _____ High: _____

DAY 27

Self-Discipline
1. Make a list of everything that you need to do today.
2. Maintain the organization of the areas that you most commonly frequent.
3. Do not allow yourself to think about anything that does not support your goals and beliefs.

Diet
1. Make a list of all the foods that you will eat today.
2. List all of the calories and carbohydrates in the meals you consume.
3. Do not exceed your daily caloric and carbohydrate allowance.

Exercise
1. Jog at least 27 minutes, then walk 3 minutes at a fast pace.
2. Start your exercise within the first hour that you are awake.
3. Drink 16 ounces of water before and after your workout.

Daily Expectations

Today you might feel challenged. You are very close to completing this program. When my clients get this close to the end of the program, they begin to go through a mourning process. For the first time in your life, you feel like you have total control over your own actions. It will only be natural for you to feel like you will miss something once you return to a normal diet plan. I want you to remember that you will always have the ability to control your body composition. I want you to maintain a disciplined diet plan when you complete this program. You need to start putting that diet plan together now. You are the one who gets to decide what you want to eat for the remainder of your life. Whether you choose a low-carbohydrate diet or a low-fat diet, the one principle remains the same: self-discipline.

If you are still a long way from having the body you have always wanted, you may want to consider maintaining a low-carbohydrate diet. The benefits of limiting your calories and carbohydrates are already more than apparent to you. I would encourage you to continue a similar eating regimen, as long as you maintain your dietary supplementation. The choice will be yours to make, because you will have the ability to eat anything you choose. You will continue to lose weight no matter what diet plan you choose.

Today I want you to develop the long-term diet plan that you will be utilizing once you have completed this program. Make sure that you factor in your tastes and preferences.

Your ketone strip should still indicate a large amount of ketones. Make sure that you monitor your breathing and complete every exercise required. Your energy might be somewhat low today due to the mourning type of effect that goes along with changing your routine. Remain focused, and remember you will always be able to control your eating habits.

Day 27

Date: _____ / _____ / _____

Daily caloric-intake limit: _____ Daily carbohydrate limit: 20

List everything that you need to accomplish today

_____

_____

_____

_____

_____

List the foods that you intend to consume today

_____

_____

_____

_____

_____

List the caloric and carbohydrate totals from the foods you consumed

Food source: _____ Caloric total: _____ Carbohydrate total: ___

Food source: _____ Caloric total: _____ Carbohydrate total: ___

Food source: _____ Caloric total: _____ Carbohydrate total: ___

Food source: _____ Caloric total: _____ Carbohydrate total: ___

Food source: _____ Caloric total: _____ Carbohydrate total: ___

Food source: _____ Caloric total: _____ Carbohydrate total: ___

Food source: _____ Caloric total: _____ Carbohydrate total: ___

Food source: _____ Caloric total: _____ Carbohydrate total: ___

Food source: _____ Caloric total: _____ Carbohydrate total: ___

Food source: _____ Caloric total: _____ Carbohydrate total: ___

Daily caloric total: _____ Daily carbohydrate total: _____

List the amount of time you were able to jog and walk

Jog: _____ Walk: _____

Place a check mark next to your current ketone level

None: _____ Trace: _____ Moderate: _____ Large: _____ High: _____

DAY 28

Self-Discipline
1. Make a list of everything that you need to do today.
2. Maintain the organization of the areas that you most commonly frequent.
3. Do not allow yourself to think about anything that does not support your goals and beliefs.

Diet
1. Make a list of all the foods that you will eat today.
2. List all of the calories and carbohydrates in the meals you consume.
3. Do not exceed your daily caloric and carbohydrate allowance.

Exercise
1. Jog at least 28 minutes, then walk 2 minutes at a fast pace.
2. Start your exercise within the first hour that you are awake.
3. Drink 16 ounces of water before and after your workout.

Daily Expectations

Today you will feel fantastic. You have developed your long-term diet plan, and you are ready to cross the finish line. I want you to turn up the energy dial today. Imagine that you have an energy dial that is numbered from 1 to 10. Today I want you to turn that energy dial to 8. Just as with every other exercise I have given you, there is a reason I am having you do this. When you imagine that you have an energy dial, you allow your mind to grasp an image that can be utilized to develop a consistent action.

Today I want you to utilize your imagination to turn up this dial. I want you to imagine that the energy dial is going to begin at 1, and turn it all the way up to 8. Once you have reached the number 8, you are going to put a lock on that number so that the number cannot decrease or increase. Tomorrow we will unlock that number and turn it up again. This use of the imagination will be a powerful tool that you will be able to utilize anytime you need an energy boost.

I want you to complete this program strong. I do not want you to feel that you have just experienced a war. You should already be over those types of feelings. You are now a very powerful individual who has great ability.

You can do anything that you set your mind to, and there is no way you could have reached this point if that were not true.

Your ketone strip should still indicate a large amount of ketones, and your energy level should be high, or you just failed this exercise. Make sure that you monitor your breathing and complete every exercise required.

Day 28

Date: _____ / _____ / _____

Daily caloric-intake limit: _____ Daily carbohydrate limit: 20

List everything that you need to accomplish today

_____

_____

_____

_____

_____

List the foods that you intend to consume today

_____

_____

_____

_____

_____

List the caloric and carbohydrate totals from the foods you consumed

Food source: _____ Caloric total: ____ Carbohydrate total: ___

Food source: _____ Caloric total: ____ Carbohydrate total: ___

Food source: _____ Caloric total: ____ Carbohydrate total: ___

Food source: _____ Caloric total: ____ Carbohydrate total: ___

Food source: _____ Caloric total: ____ Carbohydrate total: ___

Food source: _____ Caloric total: ____ Carbohydrate total: ___

Food source: _____ Caloric total: ____ Carbohydrate total: ___

Food source: _____ Caloric total: ____ Carbohydrate total: ___

Food source: _____ Caloric total: ____ Carbohydrate total: ___

Food source: _____ Caloric total: ____ Carbohydrate total: ___

Daily caloric total: _____ Daily carbohydrate total: _____

List the amount of time you were able to jog and walk

Jog: _____ Walk: _____

Place a check mark next to your current ketone level

None: _____ Trace: _____ Moderate: _____ Large: _____ High: _____

DAY 29

Self-Discipline
1. Make a list of everything that you need to do today.
2. Maintain the organization of the areas that you most commonly frequent.
3. Do not allow yourself to think about anything that does not support your goals and beliefs.

Diet
1. Make a list of all the foods that you will eat today.
2. List all of the calories and carbohydrates in the meals you consume.
3. Do not exceed your daily caloric and carbohydrate allowance.

Exercise
1. Jog at least 29 minutes, then walk 1 minute at a fast pace.
2. Start your exercise within the first hour that you are awake.
3. Drink 16 ounces of water before and after your workout.

Daily Expectations

Today I cannot express the level of energy that you are going to have. You should have gotten out of bed and jumped onto that treadmill or onto the street without a second thought. You are everything that you thought you could be. You are a day away from completing a program that some Special Forces candidates have failed!

Before we get too far into the celebration, I want you to unlock that energy dial and crank it up to 9. Lock that number in. You are to think and act as if you have an energy level of 9 out of 10. I want you to absolutely dominate any thought that goes against your beliefs. Today you are to assume total control over your life. Stay focused and vibrate with energy today. I have trained some of the fittest clients in the world, and many of them could not complete every aspect of this program. The restricted carbohydrates defeated them every time.

I have had professional athletes ask me why I have my clients jog for only thirty minutes. I told them that anyone who can jog for thirty minutes with less than twenty carbohydrates in their system is an absolute warrior. A lot of people can jog for thirty minutes, but how many can do it after restricting carbohydrates and calories from their bodies? You are less than a day away from completing a program that has been labeled the toughest fat-loss program ever developed. Congratulations! Enjoy your success, and we will start again tomorrow. I am beyond impressed with your level of ambition and dedication. You are going to succeed at anything you do in life.

You already know that you are still in ketosis. You can throw away the rest of your testing strips if you want. You are awesome!

Day 29

Date: _____ / _____ / _____

Daily caloric-intake limit: _____ Daily carbohydrate limit: 20

List everything that you need to accomplish today

_____
_____
_____
_____
_____

List the foods that you intend to consume today

_____
_____
_____
_____
_____

List the caloric and carbohydrate totals from the foods you consumed

Food source: _____ Caloric total: _____ Carbohydrate total: ___
Food source: _____ Caloric total: _____ Carbohydrate total: ___
Food source: _____ Caloric total: _____ Carbohydrate total: ___
Food source: _____ Caloric total: _____ Carbohydrate total: ___
Food source: _____ Caloric total: _____ Carbohydrate total: ___
Food source: _____ Caloric total: _____ Carbohydrate total: ___
Food source: _____ Caloric total: _____ Carbohydrate total: ___
Food source: _____ Caloric total: _____ Carbohydrate total: ___
Food source: _____ Caloric total: _____ Carbohydrate total: ___
Food source: _____ Caloric total: _____ Carbohydrate total: ___

Daily caloric total: _____ Daily carbohydrate total: _____

List the amount of time you were able to jog and walk

Jog: _____ Walk: _____

Place a check mark next to your current ketone level

None: _____ Trace: _____ Moderate: _____ Large: _____ High: _____

DAY 30

Self-Discipline
1. Make a list of everything that you need to do today.
2. Maintain the organization of the areas that you most commonly frequent.
3. Do not allow yourself to think about anything that does not support your goals and beliefs.
Diet
1. Make a list of all the foods that you will eat today.
2. List all of the calories and carbohydrates in the meals you consume.
3. Do not exceed your daily caloric and carbohydrate allowance.
Exercise
1. Jog 30 minutes, and do not dare walk at any point during your workout.
2. Start your exercise within the first hour that you are awake.
3. Drink 16 ounces of water before and after your workout.

Daily Expectations

I do not need to tell you anymore what you may feel like. Today is a day that I hope you will not ever forget. Today you get to enjoy absolutely everything you have been through over the past thirty days. Before we begin the celebration, I want you to unlock that energy dial from 9 and turn it all the way up to 10. I want you to act and think with more energy than you have had the entire program. Today is a day of power; you are now at a point in your life where you will be able to accomplish anything you want. You already know how tough it was to complete every exercise in this program.

One of the most important elements of this program is the ability to follow directions. If you successfully completed every exercise in this program, you are more than aware of the level of dedication it took to actually complete them. Every exercise you completed prepared you for the next step in this program. This program will not be complete until you complete your thirty minutes of jogging. Once you successfully complete your jog, you will join an elite class of individuals who have earned the right to say that they have completed the most intense fat-loss program ever designed. You no longer need a pat on the back for encouragement, because you are now your own best motivator.

It has been my pleasure to pass on the gifts that have been provided to me. I wish you the best in your journey to maintain peace and certainty. You have all the tools you will ever need inside of you right now. Always maintain your balance, and always remain aggressive in your pursuit for success. I can identify anyone off the street who has completed this program. The best way I can describe this level of self-discipline is to compare it to an effortless confidence that looks so easy but requires so much dedication. You did an excellent job!

Day 30

Date: _____ / _____ / _____

Daily caloric-intake limit: _____ Daily carbohydrate limit: 20

Body composition measurements

Right upper arm _____ Waistline _____ Hips _____ Right upper thigh _____

List everything that you need to accomplish today

_____

_____

_____

_____

_____

List the foods that you intend to consume today

_____

_____

_____

_____

_____

List the caloric and carbohydrate totals from the foods you consumed

Food source: _____ Caloric total: _____ Carbohydrate total: ___

Food source: _____ Caloric total: _____ Carbohydrate total: ___

Food source: _____ Caloric total: _____ Carbohydrate total: ___

Food source: _____ Caloric total: _____ Carbohydrate total: ___

Food source: _____ Caloric total: _____ Carbohydrate total: ___

Food source: _____ Caloric total: _____ Carbohydrate total: ___

Food source: _____ Caloric total: _____ Carbohydrate total: ___

Food source: _____ Caloric total: _____ Carbohydrate total: ___

Food source: _____ Caloric total: _____ Carbohydrate total: ___

Food source: _____ Caloric total: _____ Carbohydrate total: ___

Daily caloric total: _____ Daily carbohydrate total: _____

List the amount of time you were able to jog and walk

Jog: _____ Walk: _____

PART VI
Maintaining Balance for Life

MAINTAINING BALANCE FOR LIFE

Now that you have established that it is possible to have an amazing amount of self-discipline, it is time to discuss how you are going to maintain that balance. There is a certain amount of energy that is generated from control over your emotions and actions. This energy has to be maintained, or you will become out of balance.

One of the first abilities you will discover that you have is the ability to control your moods. This is done by not allowing unwanted thoughts into your mind. Throughout the entire exercise portion of this program, you were instructed to make sure that your thoughts supported your beliefs and goals. There is a deeper meaning behind the habit that you were creating in your life.

When you direct your thoughts toward the things that you want most in life, you are directing the mental energy that you have toward a constructive goal. When you are focused on a goal, you have to generate enough energy toward that goal to produce a noticeable outcome. Think about it. Why were you unable to accomplish the things that you wanted before you had self-control? The answer is that you were unable to maintain a constant flow of energy toward accomplishing that particular goal. Energy is required to accomplish any action in life. You have deprived your body of its primary fuel source for thirty days. How were you able to maintain a constant flow of energy? That energy did not come from the foods you consumed; it came from a place deep inside of you. The ability to direct energy is accomplished only when you have reached the level of self-discipline that you now have. Now that you have control over your body, it is time to direct that energy inward.

One of the first things you have to do in order to maintain balance is control your impulses. An *impulse* is a strong reaction that happens within your mind that compels you to perform a certain action or generate a certain thought. That impulse creates energy before it can produce a visible action. If you are able to stop that energy before it has a chance to gain momentum, you will be able to live a life free of impulsive behavior. This is a very advanced form of self-discipline.

When you are able to assume complete control over your impulses, you will no longer be a victim of the world around you. If you take a closer look at your behavior, you will find that you are often controlled by two driving forces: pain and pleasure. You will avoid pain at all costs, so whenever you see something that disturbs you, it creates a reaction in your mind that stimulates a response of fear. That response is now anchored within your mind and will be utilized against you at a later date.

For example: You want to start your own business, but you are afraid that you may lose a lot of time and money if it goes under. If the fear of starting your own business scares you more than the thought of how happy you will be if the business succeeds, you will act on the stronger impulse. The impulse attached to your feelings is the same impulse that creates energy within your body to create action. Therefore, instead of starting your own business, you decide to act on the stronger impulse to play it safe and avoid the risk of pain altogether. Do you see that you already experienced the feeling of pain once when you thought about losing time and money? What other pain could be experienced if you had already experienced the pain once before?

Doors are going to begin flying open for you once you find the correct answer. If you have trouble finding the answer, it may help you to go back to the section on proper breathing. When you are able to assume control over your impulses, you are assuming total control over the direction of your life. Freedom from unwanted impulses has been enjoyed by some people since the beginning of time. The ability to control an impulse comes from the same ability that you have developed over the last thirty days.

In order to control your impulses, you must first look at what you are compelled to do. If you are compelled to feel sorry for yourself, the only way to correct this problem is to begin assuming responsibility for your actions. If you are in a mental state of feeling sorry for yourself, you have to be able to correct that state. The next time you begin to feel sorry for yourself, I want you to stop in the middle of that train of thought and laugh. When you interrupt that train of thought, you are interrupting the energy that was being supplied to it.

Now that you have interrupted that flow of energy, you are free to direct that energy toward the things that you want in life. The things that you want in life can be as simple as peace and certainty. You can add more at a later time if you wish, but you have to have a place for that energy to flow. When people are depressed, they are in a mental state that allows them to think only about the negative things in their lives. You would think that it would be easy for such people to just snap out of it, but it is not that simple.

Changing a mental state requires consistent action over an extended period of time in order to develop into a habit. You should know a lot about that, considering the habits that you have broken free of over the past thirty days. Some people think that all they have to do is think happy thoughts and everything will be OK. It is not that simple. In order to break free from any unwanted habit, you have to be willing to wage an all-out war against that habit for at least thirty days.

Remember, it takes energy to direct your thoughts. If you attempt to fix every unwanted habit you have ever had all at once, you will not have the energy to successfully defeat that habit. That is why I had you focus only on your goals and beliefs for the past thirty days. I knew that if I could keep your energy directed toward one thing for at least thirty days, you would develop it into a permanent habit. When you are having negative feelings, you must be able to release the energy that is attached to them and redirect those thoughts to support your goals. This is accomplished by correcting the impulses that you have toward the negative habits.

When you are able to take away the old reaction you have had to a negative habit and replace it with certainty and confidence, you will be able to permanently eliminate that negative habit. In order to do this, you have to be willing to let go of the old emotion that you have associated with it. This requires *faith*, which is the ability to accept the unknown and just *believe*. When you have the ability to exercise faith, you will have the ability to assume total control over your own emotions. Instead of being controlled by your impulses, you will simply allow your mind to rest and not fight at all.

Most people, including myself for a great number of years, believe that if you really want something, you need to fight for it. This is true—you do have to fight for it, but it is not in the way that you might think. If someone makes a negative comment about your character or looks, you will often experience a negative reaction, which will in turn create a negatively impulsive behavior. Every time you think about that negative experience, you will experience the pain or anger all over again. I want you to pay really close attention to what I am going to share with you, because it has the ability to change your life forever if you take it seriously.

A thought is generated from a feeling, not the other way around. Most people feel that if they think of a painful experience, they will experience that painful experience all over again. The truth of the matter is that the feeling of pain is what triggered the thought to even take place. So many people feel that they are controlled by their thoughts, but they are not. They are controlled by the feelings they have associated with those thoughts. The reason I was so insistent on you directing your thoughts toward your goals and beliefs was that I wanted you to experience what happens when you mute those negative thoughts. When you are able to maintain focus, you will never have to deal with the same temptations that you would if you were to dwell on negative past experiences. Now that you have reached a level of self-discipline that will allow you to take your life to the next level, you need to begin exercising faith.

Faith is a reaction that takes place in your body when you just let go and believe you will be OK. It is also a reaction that allows you to move forward without having proof that you can see. This is very important, because the ability to pursue a goal that you cannot yet see requires faith. If you did not have faith that something would work, you would never have the energy to find out. Think about it. Would you start a fat-loss program if you did not think you would lose fat? Of course you wouldn't. Even if you felt that you would not succeed at losing fat, you would still have to have the energy within you to create the action to begin the program.

Faith is rest for your personal energy. When you have faith, you do not have to rely on yourself to accomplish everything. You allow God to take control of the ability to open doors for you. There is no way you will ever be able to have an enormous amount of personal energy if you do not utilize faith in your daily walk through life. When you say that you are going to accomplish something, how do you know that you are going to accomplish it? There is no way you can tell me for certain that you can do something. Even if you have accomplished something a million times before, there is no way that you can know for certain that you will be able to do it again. Your confidence and self-esteem both rely on faith. You can call it personal power or any other name you choose, but the fact remains the same: the only way you will ever know if you can accomplish something is when you rest on faith to make it happen. If you think that you are in total control of the world around you, you are sadly mistaken. The only thing that you will be in control of is the ability to utilize faith. Once you have the self-discipline to accomplish this, you are destined for success in all that you do.

I want to share with you an exercise that has changed my life forever, and I hope that you will utilize it to change yours as well. We will first begin with old memories, and we will work our way up from there. You started part of this exercise in the later days of the program, but you will now be able to fully capitalize on your memories. Right now, I want you to remember one really negative experience that has happened to you in your past. I want you to pay special attention to the way that you feel as you think about that memory. Remember, your feeling is what stimulated that thought. Now that you have that memory fresh in your mind, I want you to break that state and think about something that brings pleasure to your life. It could be your family, or it could be your favorite hobby. It does not matter what the pleasant memory is, as long as you focus on how good it makes you feel.

I wanted you to break that negative state because you cannot fix the impulse that is attached to the memory while you are still in the active state of that particular memory. You can change the association you have with it, but you cannot change the impulse that creates the thought attached to the feeling. Now that you are completely out of the old negative state, I want you to begin to train your ability to have faith. This is accomplished by remembering the old negative thought. Instead of having a reaction to it, just relax and let your faith take over. Instead of feeling scared, you will just relax and accept whatever happens. Your mind may tell you that there is danger if you do this, but that is a part of the fear that is driving the impulse. Make sure you utilize your breathing exercise; it will help you release the energy that is attached to the memory.

You are probably not going to be able to release all of the energy on your first attempt, but you have to remain patient and continue to recall that memory until you feel that there is no longer a negative association attached to the memory. What you want to accomplish by doing this is to back up to the point where your body first responded to the memory. Once you are on the front side of the impulse, you will be free from the impulse altogether.

The best analogy I can offer is that it is similar to a slide. You have total control of your body before you go down the slide, but after you have decided to let go of the rails, you are at the mercy of gravity. The slide is the active state of the impulse, just like in a traditional slide. If you stretch your arms and legs out wide enough, you will eventually be able to slow down to a stop. However, you will still have to climb back up that slippery slide. Imagine having to climb up a slide that is found on a playground. It is possible, but it requires a lot more energy than it does if you just let go. What we are doing with this exercise is allowing you to crawl back up that slide, so that you can get to the top, where you have control.

Some people think that if you were in total control of all your impulses, you would not be able to enjoy the pleasures in life. I thought that was true as well, until I understood that when you are the one who chooses which impulses you wish to act on, you are in control of the amount of happiness in your life. You can literally slide down any impulse you want once you have the ability to choose. This exercise is not easy, because you have to climb back up that slippery slide; however, once you persevere long enough, you will be able to get to the top.

When that happens, you will be living a life free of fear and worry, and you will be living a life full of peace and certainty. I urge you to pursue this exercise for as long as it takes to fully understand the benefits that come along with it.

I want to thank you for taking the time to experience all that you are truly capable of. This is just the tip of the iceberg of wisdom and understanding that you will gain once you understand the importance of faith. I wish you the best in your walk with faith, and I know that you will stay committed to the changes that have taken place in your life.

You would have never made it through these last thirty days if you did not have what it takes to succeed.

God bless.

Glossary

Body composition: the way in which your body's fat and muscle are composed throughout your body.

Calorie: the amount of heat required to raise the temperature of one kilogram of water one degree Celsius.

Carbohydrate: an essential nutrient that provides energy to the body. This nutrient has four calories per gram.

Cardiovascular training: a method of training that strengthens and improves the function of the heart and blood vessels.

Circuit training: a method of training that utilizes a series of different exercise stations while permitting only a brief amount of rest between each.

Continuous training: a method of training that maintains a consistent level of intensity throughout the entire exercise, such as walking and jogging.

Diet: a way of eating that is governed by a predetermined set of guidelines and parameters.

Dynamic workout: a method of training that maintains a constant or varying amount of resistance throughout the entire workout.

Exercise: the act of exerting energy toward a particular action.

Faith: the ability to believe that you can perform a desired act or receive a desired outcome without having proof.

Fat: an essential nutrient that provides energy and can be stored within the body to provide insulation and contour. This nutrient has nine calories per gram.

Interval training: intense periods of exercise that are combined with periods of less intensity within the same workout.

Ketosis: an increase in ketone bodies within the body, usually as a result of low-carbohydrate dieting or fasting.

Momentum: the force generated from the body when it is put into motion toward a desired outcome.

Mental energy: the mind's capacity to perform a desired action.

Metabolic rate: the amount of calories the body utilizes during a twenty-four-hour period.

Physical energy: the body's capacity to perform a desired action.

Self-discipline: the ability to control and direct one's own actions.

Strength training: a method of training that increases the body's muscle strength and helps prevent injury during activity.

Target heart rate: the number of heartbeats per minute required to maintain the appropriate training intensity.

VO2 max: the optimal amount of oxygen that can be consumed during activity.

Index

978-0-595-36254-7
0-595-36254-0

www.ingramcontent.com/pod-product-compliance
Lightning Source LLC
Chambersburg PA
CBHW020413290526
45785CB00002B/542